Judith L. Rozie-Battle, MSW, JD
Editor

☑ **W9-DEA-395**

African-American Adolescents in the Urban Community: Social Services Policy and Practice Interventions

African-American Adolescents in the Urban Community: Social Services Policy and Practice Interventions has been co-published simultaneously as *Journal of Health & Social Policy*, Volume 15, Number 2 2002.

Pre-publication
REVIEWS,
COMMENTARIES,
EVALUATIONS . . .

" A COMPELLING WHOLE-SYSTEMS LOOK at the realities confronting African-American youth today. . . . Includes successful strategies, practical implications, and recommendations for further action. . . . Sure to be of value to academicians, policy makers, and practitioners alike."

Elizabeth Devine Jones, MA
Consultant on Youth, Education, and Community Development, Maryland

More pre-publication
REVIEWS, COMMENTARIES, EVALUATIONS . . .

"**E**NLIGHTENING AND EMPOWERING. . . . A must read for everyone working with raising, mentoring, and in any way having significant contact with African-American adolescents. In this work of genius we have been taken beyond the 'comfort zones' and 'danger zones' of our own conditioning. Do society a great favor–read it, practice its concepts, and then share with an urban adolescent."

Abdul-Rahmann Abd-Raheem Muhammad, MSW
*Senior Vice President
and Diversity Manager
The Village for Families
and Children Inc.
Hartford, Connecticut*

"**A** COMPREHENSIVE VIEW of the challenges and opportunities that African-American youth face in today's changing society. . . . Shows that today's African-American youth face challenges that previous generations did not encounter. A MUST READ."

Michael Bonds, PhD
*Assistant Professor, Department
of Educational Policy
and Community Studies
University of Wisconsin-Milwaukee*

The Haworth Press. Inc.

African-American Adolescents
in the Urban Community:
Social Services Policy
and Practice Interventions

African-American Adolescents in the Urban Community: Social Services Policy and Practice Interventions has been co-published simultaneously as *Journal of Health & Social Policy*, Volume 15, Number 2 2002.

The *Journal of Health & Social Policy* Monographic "Separates"

Below is a list of " separates," which in serials librarianship means a special issue simultaneously published as a special journal issue or double-issue *and* as a "separate" hardbound monograph. (This is a format which we also call a "DocuSerial.")

"Separates" are published because specialized libraries or professionals may wish to purchase a specific thematic issue by itself in a format which can be separately cataloged and shelved, as opposed to purchasing the journal on an on-going basis. Faculty members may also more easily consider a "separate" for classroom adoption.

"Separates" are carefully classified separately with the major book jobbers so that the journal tie-in can be noted on new book order slips to avoid duplicate purchasing.

You may wish to visit Haworth's Website at . . .

http://www.HaworthPress.com

. . . to search our online catalog for complete tables of contents of these separates and related publications.

You may also call 1-800-HAWORTH (outside US/Canada: 607-722-5857), or Fax 1-800-895-0582 (outside US/Canada: 607-771-0012), or e-mail at:

getinfo@haworthpressinc.com

African-American Adolescents in the Urban Community: Social Services Policy and Practice Interventions, edited by Judith L. Rozie-Battle, MSW, JD (Vol. 15, No. 2, 2002). *"A comprehensive view of the challenges and opportunities that African-American youth face in today's changing society. . . . Shows that today's African-American youth face challenges that previous generations did not encounter. A must read." (Michael Bonds, PhD, Assistant Professor, Department of Educational Policy and Community Studies, University of Wisconsin-Milwaukee)*

Health and the American Indian, edited by Priscilla A. Day, MSW, and Hilary N. Weaver, DSW (Vol. 10, No. 4, 1999). *Discusses the health and mental health of Native American Indians from several aspects.*

Reason and Rationality in Health and Human Services Delivery, edited by John T. Pardeck, PhD, ACSW, Charles F. Longino, Jr., PhD, and John W. Murphy, PhD (Vol. 9, No. 4, 1998). *"A variety of perspectives that successfully challenge the pillars of modern medicine . . . . This book should be required of all health care professionals, especially those training to become physicians." (Roland Meinert, PhD, President, Missouri Association for Social Welfare, Jefferson City, Missouri)*

Selected Practical Problems in Health and Social Research, edited by Thomas E. Dinero, PhD (Vol. 8, No. 1, 1996). *"Explores some of the theoretical ideas underlying classical and modern measurement theory. These ideas form a set of guidelines for researchers, health professionals, and students in the social, psychological, or health sciences who are planning and evaluating a measurement activity." (Inquiry)*

Psychosocial Aspects of Sickle Cell Disease: Past, Present, and Future Directions of Research, edited by Kermit B. Nash, PhD (Vol. 5, No. 3/4, 1994). *"An excellent contribution to a neglected area of study and practice. . . . Offer[s] tools and techniques that one can easily incorporate into practice. Novice readers as well as seasoned practitioners will find the practicality of the book extremely helpful." (Social Work in Health Care)*

Health Care for the Poor and Uninsured: Strategies That Work, edited by Nellie P. Tate, PhD, and Kevin T. Kavanagh, MD, MS (Vol. 3, No. 4, 1992). *"Chapters are short and to the point with clearly defined goals, methods, techniques, and impacts and include easy-to-comprehend charts and statistics. This book will prove useful in understanding activities that may soon be an integral part of the American health care system." (Journal of Community Health)*

African-American Adolescents in the Urban Community: Social Services Policy and Practice Interventions

Judith L. Rozie-Battle, MSW, JD
Editor

African-American Adolescents in the Urban Community: Social Services Policy and Practice Interventions has been co-published simultaneously as *Journal of Health & Social Policy*, Volume 15, Number 2 2002.

The Haworth Press, Inc.
New York ☐ London ☐ Oxford

*African-American Adolescents in the Urban Community: Social
Services Policy and Practice Interventions* has been co-published
simultaneously as *Journal of Health & Social Policy™,* Volume 15,
Number 2 2002.

The development, preparation, and publication of this work has been undertaken with great care. However, the publisher, employees, editors, and agents of The Haworth Press and all imprints of The
Haworth Press, Inc., including The Haworth Medical Press® and Pharmaceutical Products Press®, are
not responsible for any errors contained herein or for consequences that may ensue from use of materi-
als or information contained in this work. Opinions expressed by the author(s) are not necessarily those
of The Haworth Press, Inc. With regard to case studies, identities and circumstances of individuals discussed herein have been changed to protect confidentiality. Any resemblance to actual persons, living
or dead, is entirely coincidental.

Cover design by Thomas J. Mayshock Jr.

Library of Congress Cataloging-in-Publication Data

African American adolescents in the urban community : social services policy and practice interventions /
Judith L. Rozie-Battle, editor.
      p. cm.
    "African American adolescents in the urban community: social services policy and
practice interventions has been co-published simultaneously as Journal of health &
social policy, volume 15, number 2, 2002."
    Includes bibliographical references and index.
    ISBN 0-7890-1714-8 (cloth : alk.paper)– ISBN 0-7890-1715-6 (pbk. : alk.paper)
    1. Social work with African American teenagers. 2. African American teenagers–Social
conditions. 3. Urban youth–United States–Social conditions. I. Rozie-Battle, Judith
HV3181 .A37 2002
362.7' 089–dc21

                  2002008455

Indexing, Abstracting & Website/Internet Coverage

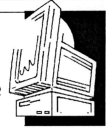

This section provides you with a list of major indexing & abstracting services. That is to say, each service began covering this periodical during the year noted in the right column. Most Websites which are listed below have indicated that they will either post, disseminate, compile, archive, cite or alert their own Website users with research-based content from this work. (This list is as current as the copyright date of this publication.)

Abstracting, Website/Indexing Coverage . . . . Year When Coverage Began

- *Abstracts in Anthropology* **1991**

- *Abstracts in Social Gerontology: Current Literature on Aging* **2000**

- *Academic Abstracts/CD-ROM* **1994**

- *AgeLine Database* **2000**

- *BUBL Information Service, an Internet-based Information Service for the UK higher education community < http://bubl.ac.uk/>* **1995**

- *c/o CAB International Access/CAB ACCESS <www.cabi.org>* **2002**

- *Cambridge Scientific Abstracts (Health & Safety Science Abstracts/Risk Abstracts) <www.csa.com>* **1990**

- *CNPIEC Reference Guide: Chinese National Directory of Foreign Periodicals* **1995**

- *EMBASE/Excerpta Medica Secondary Publishing Division <www.elsevier.nl>* **1992**

- *Family & Society Studies Worldwide <www.nisc.com>* **1996**

(continued)

- *Family Violence & Sexual Assault Bulletin* 1999

- *FINDEX <www.publist.com>* 1999

- *Health Care Literature Information Network/HECLINET* 1995

- *Health Management Information Service (HELMIS)* 1995

- *Health Source: Indexing & Abstracting of 160 selected health
  related journals, updated monthly: EBSCO Publishing* 1994

- *Health Source Plus: Expanded version of "Health Source":
  EBSCO Publishing* 1994

- *Healthcare Marketing Abstracts* 1992

- *HealthPromis* 1997

- *HealthSTAR* 1990

- *IBZ International Bibliography of Periodical Literature
  <www.saur.de>* 1996

- *Index Guide to College Journals (core list compiled
  by integrating 48 indexes frequently used to support
  undergraduate programs in small to medium sized
  libraries)* 1999

- *Index to Periodical Articles Related to Law* 1990

- *International Political Science Abstracts/Documentation
  Politique Internationale, now also available on CD/ROM
  with data from 1989 to present. Database updated
  four (4) times a year* 1992

- *Medical Benefits* 1992

- *MEDLINE (National Library of Medicine)
  <www.nlm.nih.gov>* 2000

- *NIAAA Alcohol and Alcohol Problems Science Database
  (ETOH) <http://etoh.niaaa.nih.gov>* 1994

- *OCLC Public Affairs Information Service <www.pais.org>* 1990

(continued)

- *Sage Public Administration Abstracts (SPAA)* **1991**
- *Social Services Abstracts <www.csa.com>.* **1990**
- *Social Work Abstracts <www.silverplatter.com/catalog/swab.htm>* . . **1990**
- *Sociological Abstracts (SA) <www.csa.com>* **1990**
- *UP-TO-DATE Publications* **1997**
- *World Agricultural Economics & Rural Sociology Abstracts*
  (c/o CAB Intl/CAB ACCESS) <www.cabi.org> **1993**
- *Worldwide Political Science Abstracts (formerly: Political Science*
  & Government Abstracts) <www.csa.com> **2001**

*Special Bibliographic Notes related to special journal issues
(separates) and indexing/abstracting:*

- indexing/abstracting services in this list will also cover material in any "separate" that is co-published simultaneously with Haworth's special thematic journal issue or DocuSerial. Indexing/abstracting usually covers material at the article/chapter level.
- monographic co-editions are intended for either non-subscribers or libraries which intend to purchase a second copy for their circulating collections.
- monographic co-editions are reported to all jobbers/wholesalers/approval plans. The source journal is listed as the "series" to assist the prevention of duplicate purchasing in the same manner utilized for books-in-series.
- to facilitate user/access services all indexing/abstracting services are encouraged to utilize the co indexing entry note indicated at the bottom of the first page of each article/chapter/contribution.
- this is intended to assist a library user of any reference tool (whether print, electronic, online, or CD-ROM) to locate the monographic version if the library has purchased this version but not a subscription to the source journal.
- individual articles/chapters in any Haworth publication are also available through the Haworth Document Delivery Service (HDDS).

For more information or to order
the **Journal of Health & Social Policy,**
visit http://www.haworthpressinc.com/store/product.asp?sku=J045

- or call (800) HAWORTH (in US and Canada) or
  (607) 722-5857 (outside US and Canada)

- or fax (800) 895-0582 (in US and Canada) or
  (607) 771-0012 (outside US and Canada)

For a list of related links,
visit http://www.haworthpressinc.com/store/product.asp?sku=J045

Urge your library to subscribe today!
With your library's print subscription,
the electronic edition of the journal can
be made available campus-wide to all
of the library's users!

African-American Adolescents in the Urban Community: Social Services Policy and Practice Interventions

CONTENTS

African American Youth in the New Millennium:
An Overview   1
Judith L. Rozie-Battle, MSW, JD

Youth Development: A Positive Strategy
for African American Youth   13
Judith L. Rozie-Battle, MSW, JD

The Plight of the African American Student:
A Result of a Changing School Environment   25
Sabra R. Smith, MA, EdD

Health Concerns for African American Youth   35
Stanley F. Battle, MSW, MPH, PhD

Child Support and African American Teen Fathers   45
Judith L. Rozie-Battle, MSW, JD

African American Girls and the Challenges Ahead   59
Judith L. Rozie-Battle, MSW, JD

African American Teens and the Neo-Juvenile
Justice System   69
Judith L. Rozie-Battle, MSW, JD

African American Males at a Crossroad   81
Stanley F. Battle, MSW, MPH, PhD

Index   93

ABOUT THE EDITOR

Judith L. Rozie-Battle, MSW, JD, is Assistant Professor of Social Welfare at the University of Wisconsin-Milwaukee. She has practiced social work in the areas of family therapy, child welfare and corrections. She has also practiced law in the areas of children's rights, family law and domestic violence. Professor Rozie-Battle teaches social welfare policy, community practice, child welfare and social welfare and the law. Her research focus is on family policy, with particular interests in child welfare, kinship care, minority youth, and adoption. She is co-editor of *The State of Black Milwaukee Through the Eyes of Children*, published in *The Black Teenage Parent* (Haworth) and *Urban League Review*. She is a member of the National Association of Social Workers and the Connecticut Bar Association.

African American Youth in the New Millennium: An Overview

Judith L. Rozie-Battle, MSW, JD

SUMMARY. African American youth today are facing a fast changing world of high technology and diminishing opportunities. This generation brings a new attitude and a challenging perspective to service providers and policy makers. The policies and interventions of the past may need an upgrade to meet the needs of this new generation. The issues of poverty and meaningful opportunities are important to this generation that opposes many mainstream philosophies. *[Article copies available for a fee from The Haworth Document Delivery Service: 1-800-HAWORTH. E-mail address: <getinfo@haworthpressinc.com> Website: <http://www.HaworthPress.com> © 2002 by The Haworth Press, Inc. All rights reserved.]*

KEYWORDS. Urban youth, hip-hop, youth policy

INTRODUCTION

This nation has experienced dramatic change and moved from an industrial society into a technological society at warped speed. During this period, African Americans have been provided "equal opportunity" and "equal access" to education, employment, health care, and other

---

Judith L. Rozie-Battle is affiliated with the University of Wisconsin-Milwaukee, Helen Bader School of Social Welfare.

[Haworth co-indexing entry note]: "African American Youth in the New Millennium: An Overview." Rozie-Battle, Judith L. Co-published simultaneously in *Journal of Health & Social Policy* (The Haworth Press, Inc.) Vol. 15, No. 2, 2002, pp. 1-12; and: *African-American Adolescents in the Urban Community: Social Services Policy and Practice Interventions* (ed: Judith L. Rozie-Battle) The Haworth Press, Inc., 2002, pp. 1-12. Single or multiple copies of this article are available for a fee from The Haworth Document Delivery Service [1-800-HAWORTH, 9:00 a.m. - 5:00 p.m. (EST). E-mail address: getinfo@haworthpressinc.com].

1

benefits of daily life. Despite these opportunities, for too many African Americans there remains an unequal and constant battle to obtain these benefits. This new era expects young people to have the skills necessary to function in a rapidly changing world. Young people today are expected to grow up and be productive citizens, in many instances without the necessary supports (Austin, 1996).

Each generation faces new challenges, but today's youth probably face newer and tougher challenges than those that preceded them. If success were measured by the material things available today, then this generation of African American youth would probably be viewed as far more successful than its parents' generation. However, it is clear that success is measured by more than material acquisitions.

The challenges facing the nation, and more importantly communities, are not just the education and preparation of the next generation for the technological skills necessary to compete in a global world, but also reaching out and beginning to understand why some young people are so turned off and hostile. Services must be developed that can make a difference in bringing them back into the fold. Not all young people are struggling, but for social service providers and other helping professionals, the focus is usually on those who are troubled and have rejected the "acceptable" paths to success.

Many African American youth today approach "adulthood ill prepared to become successful and active members in the community, instead they are incomplete, mistrustful, and full of fear" (Harlan, 1998). As a result, too many of these youth have become part of the "growing marginalization and isolation of the Black urban poor" (Sullivan, 1996).

THE "HIP-HOP" GENERATION

The young urban population of the 21st century has been referred to as the "hip-hop" generation. Generally, this term refers to the culmination of a music form (rap), clothing fashions, and a general in-your-face life style. The influence of this urban hip-hop culture has extended beyond the inner city into suburban as well as international communities. So despite the negative images the general adult population sees in this life style, youth of all races and economic backgrounds are attracted to various aspects of the hip hop lifestyle.

Unfortunately, "significant numbers of Black youth have developed an alternative means of validating themselves, adopting a core of 'oppositional' or 'gangsta' norms that they associate with being authentically Black" (Brown, 2000). The issue is how to provide guidance and support to help these young people mature and develop into productive adults. The task is not easy for youth who are so turned off to the mainstream and view successful African Americans as "sell outs" to the rest of the community. They view rap stars, with "thug" mentalities, as their heroes and belittle their colleagues who work hard to achieve academic success.

A number of sociological theories have been advanced to explain the level of violence that appears to be so prevalent among African American youth. These include: genetic inferiority, culture of poverty, and racial oppression/discrimination. To explain each theory briefly, the genetic inferiority theory states that African Americans have an innate proclivity toward aggression and consequently commit crimes; the culture of poverty theory states that poor families and community values result from a poverty that allows antisocial behavior; and, finally, the racial discrimination theory states that African American crime is the result of racism by the dominant group in society. Regardless of which theory is advanced, the consequence is the alienation of many youth from the general society (Schiele, 1998). This resulting alienation is instrumental in shaping the antisocial behavior prevalent in too many African American urban youth.

There are many tensions pulling young people, including violence in their schools and communities, the pervasive violence in rap, music videos, video games, and the persistent violence in the mass media. These mediums have often been criticized for the violence and lack of respect toward women and violence toward others in general. Exposure to violence on television over long periods of time can impact individuals in the following ways: they can become less sensitive to the pain and suffering of others; they can exhibit more fear of the world around them; they are more likely to behave aggressively toward others; and they are more prone to think aggressive behavior is normal (Silverblatt, 1995). The existence of a market for these products is a symptom of broader societal ills.

The hostility and refusal to participate in the traditional roles expected of young adults cannot be squarely placed on the exposure to violence alone. Despite the fact that African American youth share the same hopes and aspirations of other community members, the lives of many African American adults and adolescents have been marked by various levels of failure (Snell and Thomas, 1998).

Issues of institutional racism remain a concern for the Black community overall. The indications are that policies regarding individual rights and equal opportunities are moving in a new direction. The political environment has begun to close the door of opportunity to all but the highest achievers. The youth of today are cognizant of these trends and believe that these efforts are aimed directly at them. Questions have been raised, particularly by young people, about the value and potency of the civil rights advocacy efforts, as the nation has moved toward more "racial intolerance, the renewal of states rights, and the dismantling of the government's protective domestic social policies and programs" (Sullivan, 1996).

It can be argued that African American youth have developed an "oppositional culture," which emphasizes respecting the values that the larger society denigrates and denigrating the values the larger society prizes (Anderson, 1994). Rather than blame young people for the declining conditions in the inner city—"the eclipse of Black civil society" has more to do with the institutional collapse of the inner city and the failure of Black social and civic organizations to empower the most isolated members of the community (Sullivan, 1996). Still other researchers believe that the "instability and hopelessness [of many poor adolescents] has caused them to develop a criminal behavior instead of positive meaningful ways to acquire the American dream" (Harlan, 1998).

This paper will now examine a few of the overriding issues that affect African American youth in the new millennium. The areas that will be addressed include: poverty, family structure and supports, community violence, child welfare, and education.

POVERTY

Despite an increase in employment rates of low-income Black adults and Black parents from 1997-1999, poverty rates remained unchanged (Staveteig and Wigton, 2000). The gap between the percentages of Blacks and Whites with low incomes increased between 1996 and 1998. In fact, the U.S. Census Bureau indicates that Black married couples are less likely than their White counterparts to have an annual income of $50,000 or more.

The African American rate of participation in the workforce is lower than that of Whites, 12% and 74%, respectively. It is also important to note that the unemployment rate for Blacks is more than twice that of Whites (McKinnon and Humes, 2000).

As a consequence of the dismal labor data, the poverty rate for Blacks is 26% as compared to the national rate of 13% and only 8% for Whites. In 1998, the poverty rate for children under 18 in this nation was approximately 19%, but the Black poverty rate was 37%, despite the fact that the population of African children and youth between the ages of 0-17 was only 15.3% of the population. As of 1998, children and youth between the ages of 0-17 comprised 35.4% of the population below 100% of the poverty level and 63.5% below 200% of the poverty level. Those children between the ages of 0-17 covered by health insurance ranged from 18% being uninsured to 49% having Medicaid/SCHIP State coverage in 1999. Approximately 30% of African American families had employer-sponsored health coverage (McKinnon and Humes, 2000).

FAMILY STRUCTURE AND SUPPORTS

In 1999, African American families accounted for 8.4 million of the families in the United States. Yet, less than one-half were married-couple families, and 45% were headed by women with no spouse present. Another 8% were headed by men with no spouse present (McKinnon and Humes, 2000). These stark percentages regarding family structure point out the dilemmas that African American parents must face, particularly the large number of single parents.

Traditionally, African American families had vast extended family networks in the same community. These family members provided a sense of support and encouragement. The other traditional source of support and guidance has been the Black church. In a study that looked at help-seeking behavior patterns for mental health services, African Americans sought help from ministers (church) first and then schools (Neighbors and Jackson, 1996). The concept of extended families has to some extent been lost, due in part to the mobility of families. Drug and alcohol addiction have also had a negative impact on the concept of the nuclear family. As a result, this negative impact has dramatically changed the traditional roles and relationships of the extended family.

In 1998, 5.4 million children lived in households headed by a relative other than a parent, 39 percent of these children–2.1 million–lived in these households with no parent present. Two-thirds of these children, or 1.4 million, lived in households headed by a grandparent (Census

Bureau, 1998). Consequently, youth turn to other resources that have replaced the family.

For some young people, peer groups and youth gangs are essentially performing the functions traditionally provided by the church and elders in the community. The alienation experienced by some youth may not be understood by their families, consequently the gang becomes the "substitute" or "surrogate" family, as well as the primary youth cohort group (Davis, 1999). These sub groups provide the support, encouragement, and guidance that adolescents naturally seek. Unfortunately, too often the guidance is directed toward negative or illegal behaviors with broader social consequences. The increase in the opportunities for drug trafficking and easy money, along with the decline in manufacturing jobs, provides reason to reject traditional routes to success for young people in the inner city (Wilson, 1987). The choice for gang involvement "reflects weak community, neighborhood, and family structures" (Davis, 1999).

COMMUNITY VIOLENCE

Reports have been widespread in the media illustrating the inability to escape violence in homes, schools, and even churches. The nation has watched in horror over the past several years the school shootings in Colorado, Georgia, Arkansas, Kentucky, California, and Michigan. The recent shootings in Texas that occurred at a church youth meeting have made it clear that no place can provide a sanction from violence.

Domestic violence is also a concern in the African American community, as it is in all communities. Too many African American children are suffering from the consequences of witnessing violence in their homes and in their communities. The devastating effects on children include Post Traumatic Stress Disorder (PTSD), regression into earlier stages of development for younger children, or self-destructive or high-risk behaviors for adolescents (Richters and Martinez, 1993; Singer, Anglin, Song, and Lunghofer, 1995). The end results are youth that are not as productive and healthy as they could be and who may begin to repeat the patterns they have been exposed to over time.

CHILD WELFARE

The overrepresentation of African American children in the juvenile court system is well documented (Snyder and Sickmund, 1999). Despite reports of decreases in the number of youth involved in delinquency cases, more serious crimes has increased, and similar to the adult system, juvenile crime statistics indicate an overrepresentation of African American youth. According to the 1990 Census, the juvenile population in this country was about 80% white and 20% minority. However, only 31% of the juvenile in public facilities were white, while 69% were African American.

Federal legislation, including the mandates of the Personal Responsibility and Work Opportunity Reconciliation Act of 1996 (PRWORA) and the Adoption and Safe Families Act of 1997 (ASFA) have played a significant role in the increase of children entering the child welfare system today. The intervention and treatment of African American children and youth in the child welfare system has been plagued by inequitable policies, insufficient services, and inadequate interventions (Billingsley, 1988). This issue is critically important to the African American community because the numbers of African American children in the system continue to soar. Black children are significantly overrepresented among abuse and neglect victims, which is more than double their proportion in the national population (Children's Bureau, 1999).

Foster care, a component of the child welfare system, has seen steady growth in the number of children placed through out-of-home care, with African American children and youth accounting for the vast majority of those in care. A record 547,000 children were reported to be in foster care as of March 31, 1999–a 35 percent increase from 1990. Sixty percent of the children in foster care are children of color; 43 percent of whom are African American (Children's Bureau, 2000).

Kinship care has become a less expensive and in some cases a less formal alternative for the placement of children when they must be removed from their homes. As of 1998, more than two million children in the United States were in some form of kinship care arrangement, of which about 10% or 200,000 were foster children (Boots and Green, 1999).

These facts demonstrate the poor state of many African American youth. The decrease in the number of nuclear family units and the increase in extended family units are common. For too many African American youth, they are caught in a system that has historically been unable to effectively care for and develop them into adulthood.

EDUCATION

Education is seen by most Americans as the major vehicle for both individual and collective progress (Holland and Russell, 1999). This nation defines success in terms of the ability to work and provide for self and family. The level of educational attainment has been one of the barometers of potential income. Clearly, some African American young people are succeeding, in the areas of higher education, as reflected in the 1.5 million African American students enrolled in colleges and universities in 1997 (The Chronicle Almanac, 2001).

However, other numbers also indicate that too few are succeeding. The African American community should be concerned when the national school drop out rate is approximately 10%, while drop out rates for African American students in some cities exceed 50%. The data also indicates that 63% of the African American college students are female, while only 37% are male (The Chronicle Almanac, 2001).

Similar proportions of African American men and women 25 years of age and older are at least high school graduates. However, African American women are more likely than African American men to have completed at least a bachelor's degree (McKinnon and Humes, 2000). As the data indicate, this gap will continue to widen as fewer and fewer young men are completing high school, let alone obtaining their college degrees. As the gap widens, it is clear that more women will be the major income earners in their families, either as single parents or as part of two-parent working families.

These issues are effecting the African American community as a whole, but more importantly they are part of the message to youth, particularly males, that there is no place for them. Arguably, if one can run fast, jump high, and handle a ball well, there will be doors opened through athletics. However, even those opportunities are limited as universities and the National Collegiate Athletic Association (NCAA) develop higher standards and entrance requirements for athletes. For the talented few who are unable to pursue higher education, the professional sports leagues are beckoning with promises of wealth and glory.

As the standards continue to rise, it is important that African American youth understand that the opportunities are narrowing and they must devote more positive efforts toward their education. The negative attitudes by some African American youth may be attributed to their adoption of the oppositional attitude that includes "the rejection of mainstream opportunity-enhancing behaviors such as educational achievement . . ." (Brown, 2000). New approaches and programs will need to be developed to attract today's youth, including programs that assist and encourage youth with their achievement.

In an effort to address the past failures of African American students to access and succeed in college, many colleges and universities have adopted a variety of pre-college programs that expose African American youth to college and prepare them for success. A large number of these programs are geared toward a wide range of youth–not just the high achievers. Examples of these program include Talent Search, Gear Up, Upward Bound, academic opportunity centers, and numerous other pre-college programs aimed at assisting youth with college readiness. These program not only serve high school students, but also reach out to elementary and middle school students with programs during both the summer and academic year.

The gap between entrance exam scores for African Americans and Whites has been discussed for many years. The scores of 1997 college bound seniors taking the Scholastic Aptitude Test (SAT) and the ACT Assessment (ACT) demonstrated that a large gap remains between the two groups. For example, for White students the average verbal score was 527 and the average math score was 524. For African Americans, the scores were 484 and 442, respectively. On the ACT, Whites averaged 21.8 while African Americans averaged 17.0 (The Chronicle Almanac, 2000-2001).

IMPLICATIONS

These issues highlight the potential obstacles that will prevent African American youth from achieving their dreams and having a successful future in the mainstream of society. Rather than being turned off the style and "attitude," policy makers and service providers will need to work to better understand the youth. If too many young people continue to be turned off to the mainstream avenues of success and achievement, then there will be a reason for concern. There will be more of the negative behaviors that are feared and less of the positive behaviors that are desired. Every youthful generation has its opposition or its resistance from the older generations, but perhaps this generation with its' swagger and "attitude" seem a bit more scary than previous generations.

Issues of poverty and family structure are intertwined. Until African American youth have fair and equal access to employment and the opportunities to learn new skills, the cycle will continue into the next generation. Another related issue is that of educational opportunities. Alternative educational programs that have more relevance for young people should be examined. Career to work program are on the rise and can be an avenue for change. Many school districts are utilizing charter and magnet schools as alternative options, but may need to go even further. Educational programs may need to gear more toward the job market to ensure that African American youth are prepared to step into the available jobs.

It may be time to seriously review and alter the policies of the child welfare and juvenile justice system, which have an overwhelmingly high representation of African American youth. Despite laws to the contrary, poverty is an underlying cause for the removal of children from their homes, and is certainly a major obstacle in the reunification of children with their families. The hope and despair of too many parents who have turned to drugs and alcohol are indicative of what the future holds if this nation is not willing to closely examine current policies and interventions as it relates to families, youth, and poverty.

Current juvenile justice policies may easily perpetuate beliefs by African American youth that no matter what they do, they will end up in "the system." They are aware of too many family members, friends, and neighbors for whom this has been the case, and currently there are few programs and services that are telling them it can be any different.

CONCLUSION

This is a new generation, that is perhaps not really that different from previous "rebellious" youthful cohorts. Although each generation faces new challenges, this generation more so than any other is faced with the unique challenges of high technology and an interactive world. They must learn skills that their parents were not exposed to and which consequently places them in a different sphere than their elders. The knowledge is available, but too many youth are anticipating obstacles and not reaching out to capture the opportunities, and it is those youth who raise the most concern. They must be reached and supported in their efforts to develop.

African American youth today desire assistance in the development of the skills that will be necessary for them to feel as though they are part of the community and to become more positive productive citizens. It is up to the adults of the African American community and the general population to be sure they receive the supports they need. The opportunity to work with young people begins with understanding the predicament they see themselves in and assisting them in learning positive approaches to overcoming these obstacles.

As the minority population grows and eventually becomes the majority, these young people today will be our leaders tomorrow. Despite the fashions, the music, and the language–they are the future.

REFERENCES

Adoption and Safe Families Act. (1997). P. L. 105-89.

Anderson, E. (1994). The code of the streets. *Atlantic Monthly.* May 1994.

Austin, B.W. (1996). *Repairing the breach.* Village Foundation. Dillon, CO: Alpine Guild, Inc.

Billingsley, A. (1988). The impact of technology on Afro-American families. *Family Relations,* October, 1988.

Boots, S. and Green, R. (1999). *Family care or foster care? How state policies affect kinship caregivers.* Report of the Assessing the New Federalism Project funded by Series A, No. A-34, The Urban Institute.

Brown, E. (2000). Black like me? "Gangsta" culture, Clarence Thomas, and Afrocentric academies. *New York University Law Review,* 75(20):308-353.

Census Bureau. (1998). Current population reports. *Marital status and living arrangements: March 1998 update.* (P20-5124) Washington, DC: U.S. Government Printing Office.

Children's Bureau. (1999). *Child maltreatment 1997: Reports from the states to the National Child Abuse and Neglect data system,* Washington, DC: Administration for Children and Families, U.S. Department of Health and Human Services.

Children's Bureau (2000). *The AFCARS report, current estimates as of January 2000.* Washington, DC: Administration for Children and Families, U.S. Department of Health and Human Services.

Davis, N. (1999). *Youth crisis growing up in the high risk society.* Westport, CT: Praeger.

Harlan, V. T. (1998). *Urban decay: Adolescent separatism, rap culture, and media.* Bethesda, MD: Winfield and Austin Publishers.

Holland, A. and Russell, R. (2000). Academic achievements and standards in the African-American community. In S. F. Battle (Ed.). *The State of Black Milwaukee,* Milwaukee, WI: Milwaukee Urban League, Inc.

McKinnon, J. and Humes, K. (2000). The Black population in the United States; March 1999, U.S. Census Bureau. *Current population reports survey P20-530.* Washington, DC: U.S. Government Printing Office.

Neighbors, H.W. and Jackson, J.S. (1996). Mental health in Black America psychosocial problems and help seeking behavior. In H.W. Neighbors and J.S. Jackson (Eds.). *Mental health in Black America.* Thousand Oaks, CA: Sage.

Richter, J. and Martinez, P. (1993). The NIMH community violence project: Children as victims of and witnesses to violence. *Psychiatry,* 56, 7-21.

Schiele, J.H. (1998). Cultural alignment, African American male youths, and violent crime. In See (Lee), L. A. Human behavior in the social environment: An African American perspective, *Journal of Human Behavior in the Social Environment,* 1(2/3).

Silverblatt, A. (1995). *Media literacy: Keys to interpreting media messages.* Westport, CT: Praeger.

Singer, M. I., Anglin, T. M., Song, L. Y., and Lunghofer, L. (1995). Adolescent exposure to violence and associated symptoms of psychological trauma. *Journal of American Medical Association,* 273(6), 477-482.

Snell, C. L. and Thomas, J.S. (1998). Young African American males: Promoting psychological and social well-being. In See (Lee), L. A. Human behavior in the social environment: An African American perspective, *Journal of Human Behavior in the Social Environment*, 1(2/3).

Synder, H. N. and Sickmund, M. (1999). *Juvenile offenders and victims:1999 national report*. Washington, DC: Office of Juvenile Justice and Delinquency Prevention, U.S. Department of Justice.

Staveteig, S. and Wigton, A. (2000). Snapshots of America's families II. Report of the Assessing the New Federalism Project, Washington, DC: Urban Institute.

Sullivan, L. Y. (1996). The demise of black civil society: Once upon a time when we were colored meets the hip hop generation. *Social Policy*, Winter.

The Chronicle of Higher Education. (2001). *The almanac of higher education: 2000-2001*.

Wilson, W.J. (1987). *The truly disadvantaged*. Chicago: University of Chicago Press.

Youth Development:
A Positive Strategy
for African American Youth

Judith L. Rozie-Battle, MSW, JD

SUMMARY. The concept of positive youth development has been discussed and implemented for over ten years. The more recent emphasis on the connection between community and youth development is as important to the African American community in general as it is to African American youth. Opportunities to experience responsibility and involvement in their community, under the guidance of supportive adults, provide youth the chance of success for themselves and, ultimately, their communities. *[Article copies available for a fee from The Haworth Document Delivery Service: 1-800-HAWORTH. E-mail address: <getinfo@haworthpressinc.com> Website: <http://www.HaworthPress.com> © 2002 by The Haworth Press, Inc. All rights reserved.]*

KEYWORDS. Positive youth development, African American youth, community development

THE IMPORTANCE OF YOUTH DEVELOPMENT

During the 1990s, the nation experienced many challenges with its youth and in its communities. The increased level of violence that per-

---

Judith L. Rozie-Battle is affiliated with the University of Wisconsin-Milwaukee, Helen Bader School of Social Welfare.

[Haworth co-indexing entry note]: "Youth Development: A Positive Strategy for African American Youth." Rozie-Battle, Judith L. Co-published simultaneously in *Journal of Health & Social Policy* (The Haworth Press, Inc.) Vol. 15, No. 2, 2002, pp. 13-23; and: *African-American Adolescents in the Urban Community: Social Services Policy and Practice Interventions* (ed: Judith L. Rozie-Battle) The Haworth Press, Inc., 2002, pp. 13-23. Single or multiple copies of this article are available for a fee from The Haworth Document Delivery Service [1-800-HAWORTH, 9:00 a.m. - 5:00 p.m. (EST). E-mail address: getinfo@haworthpressinc.com].

meated rural, suburban, and urban communities has been documented and visualized nightly on local newscasts. A number of factors, including the increase in drug use among parents and young people, increased gang involvement, teen parenthood, and the overall violence in many communities are destroying the ability of communities to grow and prosper. Despite the economic prosperity of much of the country, many inner city neighborhoods continue to experience stymied growth.

Teens, those between the ages of 12 and 18, are particularly affected by the challenges presented in urban communities. This same group of young people are also dropping out of school at astonishing rates, particularly African American and other minority students. Standardized exams indicate lower scores for students of color, regardless of economic status (The College Board, 1999).

To alleviate some of the challenges presented, a number of programs have been developed in schools and community-based organizations. These programs include violence prevention, peer leadership, conflict resolution, cultural awareness, tutoring, and substance abuse education. A growing number of after school programs and activities have been developed that focus on adolescents, not just younger children. Philanthropic supporters and national youth organizations such as: DeWitt Wallace Reader's Digest Fund, The Center for Youth Development, Search Institute, The Center for Early Adolescence, the Mott Foundation, and The Carnegie Council on Adolescent Development have looked at services to youth and the effectiveness of existing programs. These groups have also raised concerns that "quick fix it" programs were not indicating long-term successes (Pittman, Irby, and Ferber, 2000). What was needed were programs that provided young people with the self confidence and skills needed to succeed as adults.

Many people are familiar with the phrase, "children are our future." While many policy makers, community leaders, and social service providers may agree with this ideology–they are generally more in agreement with this phrase when the term "children" refers to preadolescent children. As a nation, there is more comfort raising concerns about young children on issues of brain development, the effects of lead poisoning, early childhood education, and the transition from preschool into kindergarten and first grade. In return, financial support for research and services to support improvement efforts in these areas has followed. Funding from both the private and public sector has increased over the past decade. Overall, most policy makers and service providers have begun to focus on early intervention. One need only to review the level of financial support from local United Ways, community foundations, and other private supporters to understand that the vast majority of funding is for programs and services to children is allocated for those under the age of 13.

Adolescents are not a popular group. As part of their normal developmental process they provide us with challenges we are not always willing nor patient enough to endure.

While early intervention is important and most would agree that prevention is the direction that health, education, and social service programming should work toward, the current adolescent population and its needs cannot be ignored. These young people between the ages of 12 and 18 are in fact the next generation of leaders. The thinking of those who consider this a "lost" generation and consequently desire to focus on only children twelve years of age and younger, cannot be accepted.

Socially competent adolescents have a sense of belonging, feel valued, and have opportunities to contribute to society through their schools, neighborhoods, and the broader society (Gullotta, 1990). Adolescents need to have real opportunities to develop and explore their capacities. They need support from parents, adults, and communities. Absent these supports and adult advisors, young people will fail, and ultimately, the nation will fail.

Efforts to strengthen this cohort of youth and their capabilities need to go beyond the local neighborhood, city, state, or even the country. With increased reliance on technology, the concept of a global world is no longer just rhetoric. Interactions and negotiations with people from throughout the world will be the norm. Youth need to be prepared to venture into this world as confidently and effectively as possible.

In a 1992 publication, *A Matter of Time*, James Comer was quoted as follows:

> Our country's family policy continues to place most of the responsibility for the raising and rearing of children on the parent or parents with whom they reside. And yet, these parents are increasingly unavailable to these children. . . . Just as families have changed so have communities. The supportive and protective functions of neighborhoods–two subtle but essential functions–have been lost for many of America's youth. (Carnegie Council on Adolescent Development, 1992)

Unfortunately, this is more true for many urban families who are plagued by drug and alcohol abuse and an overrepresentation in the juvenile and child welfare systems. Extended family, community based organizations, after-school programs, and church activities have become critical replacements to meet the basic emotional and developmental needs of many youth. For those young people unable to make connections with family or the other critical replacements mentioned, the streets and gangs become the source for meeting their basic emotional and developmental needs.

YOUTH DEVELOPMENT

The phrase "positive youth development" (PYD) was developed and implemented by youth oriented advocates in the early 1990s. PYD focused on providing supports and opportunities to assist young people to develop into successful and engaged adults. The movement focused on emphasizing the positive assets of young people as opposed to the negative attributes. Several components are key: ongoing positive relationships with adults and other youth, active involvement in community life, and availability of positive choices for young people to participate in during their non-school hours (Walker, 2000).

Research supports the thinking that a strengths focused approach to adolescent development is useful in helping improve the outlook and confidence of young people (Carnegie Council on Adolescent Development, 1992; Scales and Leffert, 1999) and reducing high-risk behaviors (Quinn, 1995).

"Youth development, when it is successful, creates a plethora of non-events–young people not using drugs, not dropping out of school, not breaking the law, not getting pregnant, and not illiterate. Although this state of non-events is what we desire, we seldom see these non-events on the evening news or in the newspaper headlines" (Dunkle, 1997). Too often we highlight the crime and violence perpetrated by a small number of youth, yet the young people involved in this negative behavior have become the poster children for all African American youth. Young African American youth are achieving at greater heights than ever before in this nation. Yet, for many people, the images they see in the newspapers, on the nightly news, in movies, and on television emphasize the stereotypes of inner city, poor, and out of control youth.

The majority of the current research on African American youth also focuses on the negative as opposed to the positive. For example, if 20% of the children under 18 in this country are in poverty, than 80% are not; if 12% of the teens are victims of crime then 88% are not; if 15% are teen parents, then 85% are not; and if 14% are high school drop outs than 86% are not. PYD looks toward the assets and strengths of youth and provides programs with an opportunity to develop services and supports that direct youth toward these outcomes.

The PYD concept requires youth providers an opportunity to re-assess how they provide services that assure that young people develop the social, emotional, cognitive, and moral competencies necessary to become productive adults. This is not always an easy transition for service providers who have never utilized this approach. For many service providers, it is difficult to allow for high levels of participation by youth in the decision-making and implementation of programs and services. Yet, this approach is one of the few ways for youth to develop new skills and knowledge and to demonstrate their abilities.

IMPORTANCE OF A YOUTH DEVELOPMENT FOR THE AFRICAN AMERICAN COMMUNITY

Historically, the positive youth development approach focused on enhancing and promoting the strengths of youth, individually and collectively. In more recent years, the approach has broadened to include the concept of community development. This expanded approach partners youth and community development to combat the negative effects of some urban communities, such as high crime, substance abuse, unemployment, and high drop out rates.

It is critical in African American communities that young people feel a sense of belonging and a pride in their respective communities. As they develop and mature into young adults there will be a higher likelihood of them remaining in the community and becoming involved in efforts to continue its improvement.

PYD programming does not necessarily need to replace existing youth oriented efforts and programming in community based organizations, schools, and churches. Instead, it seeks to change the attitude and method of approaching the development of our youth by pushing them to expand their capabilities and horizons to achieve whatever goals they establish for themselves. These skills and attitudes can be incorporated into current youth programming in any community.

Social competence is facilitated through supportive relationships and a supportive socioeconomic environment, while the inhibitors of social competence include cultural and social barriers based upon factors such as race and socioeconomic status (Bloom, 1990). For African American youth who have historically been discouraged, disenfranchised, and turned off to many programs and services, it allows them to have more input into the types of programs they desire. Another important aspect of this approach for the African American community is that it does not focus only on the high achievers and college bound youth. It is inclusive to all youth, and perhaps more concerned about the youth who are perceived as non-college bound and have fallen through the cracks in the past. A youth development approach seeks to capture the youth who has not already been labeled as a troubled child and who may not be perceived as an outstanding student in their community (Pittman, Irby, and Ferber, 2000). With proper implementation, these youth can be encouraged to pursue their dreams and build their self-confidence.

There are a number of successful programs operating in the nation that exemplify the concepts of youth development. For example, the National Urban League's Incentives To Excel and Succeed, (NULITES) program is a nationwide initiative designed to reflect the positive aspects of urban youth while providing opportunities for personal development and leadership in local communities. Activities are developed, implemented, and executed by youth participants with guidance from adult advisors. NULITES has developed an annual conference that focuses on preparing young people to be self-sufficient, competent and contributing members of society and their communities (National Urban League, 2001). This program exemplifies the connection between youth development and community development.

Another example is the After-School Initiative (ASI) operating in Hartford, Connecticut, and funded by the Hartford Foundation for Public Giving. This initiative began as a opportunity for youth serving organizations to receive financial resources to support their program efforts with youth. ASI was an effort, on the part of a community foundation, to develop a network of youth serving programs that utilized the positive youth development ideology. Through its first five years, ASI allocated financial and technical assistance to fourteen different youth serving organizations, and was instrumental in developing an infrastructure in the City of Hartford for youth development programming (Meister, 1999).

Finally, an example from Milwaukee, Wisconsin, is the Strive Media Institute (Strive). Strive was founded in 1990, as a non-profit organization located in the city of Milwaukee. It provides mentoring and hands-on training to metropolitan area teens interested in mass communications. Strive helps expose and prepare a diverse group of youth with the skills necessary to pursue a career in the communications field. Strive's program has real life outcomes in the form of two TV shows (Teen Forum and GTV), a nationally distributed teen magazine (GUMBO), a computer consulting program (TechKnow), and an annual Media Summit Conference (Strive Media Institute, 2001).

The keys to the success of a program such as Strive are the involvement of caring adult mentors on the staff. These young people are actually given the opportunity to make decisions about what they publish, what is aired, and the development of websites, among many other responsibilities. The youth conduct the research and the interviews for the television show and the magazine. They also write and edit the articles and the scripts. Through their involvement in Strive, a number of the youth are asked to participate in other community events, such as anti-tobacco and anti-violence efforts. They begin to take on real responsibilities, not only in the work at Strive, but also in the wider community. This program also exemplifies the dual approach to youth and community development.

POLICY RECOMMENDATIONS/IMPLICATIONS

There are a number of issues in the field of youth development that must be addressed if services and outcomes for youth and their respective communities are to improve. Pittman discusses a paradigm shift in the approach to services for youth. There must be a continued and broadened shift in the goals to promote problem reduction for adolescents, increase options for involvement, and a re-definition of strategies "to ensure a broad scale of supports and opportunities for young people that reach beyond the status quo" (Pittman, Irby, and Ferber, 2000).

There is a need for a comprehensive approach to reaching adolescents and helping them develop into successful adults. In order to avoid unsuccessful, short-term strategies, policy makers and funders need to provide resources which foster long-term programming and services for children and youth. Currently, the federal government provides support for a number of prevention programs during the preschool and elementary school years. The federal government currently supports Head Start for preschool children. Additional support is also available for transition programs in early education and prevention efforts are funded for school-age children through after-school activities. Increased funding is necessary for teens in the middle through high school years. This continuity in funding would provide the long-term supports necessary to ensure all children and youth, particularly those that are disadvantaged, with the developmental supports necessary for transition into adulthood.

Organizations such as the National Urban League have focused on the needs of adolescents through its Education and Youth Development Policy, Research and Advocacy program. Programs similar to this one need to be financially supported nationally. In addition, there must be efforts to revive the Youth Development Community Block Grant Bill (HR 2807) to allocate resources for services to youth, particularly older adolescents.

There must be a focus on the cohort of young people in the middle through high school years. This is a group that with appropriate adult involvement, positive activities, and good peer relationship can achieve a number of successes. In general, they will remain in school, they will graduate, they will not be involved in the criminal justice system, and they will not become parents before they reach adulthood. Studies indicate that all of the outcomes listed will be more positive for the young person who feels confident and supported (Gambone, 1997; Dunkle, 1997; Roehlkepartain and Benson, 1996).

The importance of providing after school as well as weekend activities to fill the time with positive activities is supported. Research findings state that juvenile violence peaks in the after school hours on school days between 3-4 p.m. and in the evenings on non-school days (Carnegie Council on Adolescent Development, 1992). The potential for reducing community juvenile violence is far greater if efforts are put into reducing after school crime than imposing juvenile curfews (Synder and Sickmund, 1999).

An effort to increase the professionalism and strengthen perceptions of youth work and youth workers through certification and increased salaries must be seriously considered. The salaries for youth workers are generally low, staff turnover is high, and credentialing is sporadic. Organizations such as the Academy for Educational Development have moved in the direction of providing training and certifications in the area of youth development. The University of Wisconsin-Milwaukee, with support from the DeWitt Wallace-Readers Digest Fund, has developed a Youth Development Certificate program, which focuses on core competencies of youth development (University of Wisconsin-Milwaukee, 2001). These are a few examples of the efforts to elevate the status of the field of youth work. More community colleges and universities should provide certifications or minors through their liberal arts curriculum, schools of social work, or human services departments. If the factor of consistent adult relationships is critical, as the research indicates, than efforts have to be made to ensure adequate income in order to attract and retain quality youth workers. The bottom line is that funders need to seriously evaluate the value of adults working with youth and allocate appropriate levels of funding to support these efforts.

For the African American community, the Black church is a vital partner in youth development. Recent studies indicate that the Black church and religious involvement for African American adolescents has a positive impact in assisting youth with positive psychosocial development (Markstrom, 1999) and that these religious institutions significantly buffer or interact with the effects of neighborhood disorder on crime, and, in particular serious crime (Johnson, Jeng et al., 2000).

Community service is an important component of youth development and should be encouraged among all youth. Traditionally, community service has been seen as an alternative to jail for those involved in the juvenile and criminal justice systems. However, in recent years a number of high schools and universities have incorporated community service into their curriculums as a requirement for graduation. A newer form of service is being developed through service learning components instituted by some colleges and universities. This option can also be developed for high school students as a requirement for graduation. For African American students, these structured activities provide opportunities for positive involvement within their own community that they may not have been aware of. Youth volunteer work experiences allows them to learn new skills, make contributions to the community, and enhance social skills, self-esteem, self-confidence, and learning capabilities.

The role of a caring adult can not be taken too lightly. The increase in mentoring programs, such as the Sullivan-Spaights Boys to Men Mentoring Institute currently operating in Milwaukee, Wisconsin, and other efforts to utilize adults in reaching children and youth is evident. Big name organizations such as, Big Brothers/Big Sisters, continue to receive positive evaluation of the outcomes they seek to achieve (Freedman, 1992). National efforts such as America's Promise, headed by Colin Powell, prior to his joining the current Bush Administration, is an example of a high profile person joining in the effort to work with children and youth. This effort focused on increasing the number of volunteers involved with youth and mentoring. The ongoing encouragement of adult involvement is critical, however, the presence of adult mentors does not preclude parental involvement with youth. It is a real partnership between parents, other adults, and the community.

The media must examine its role in the effort to develop youth and profile the positive side of this generation. Not only must the media highlight constructive activities and services that African American youth are involved with, they must also encourage youth involvement through the development of local teen advisory boards. These advisory boards could provide input on teens' interests and needs with such entities as local media, libraries, city planning, recreation departments, and health centers, to name a few. These advisory boards would provide teens with the opportunity to be involved in the community and to have their voices heard.

Finally, there is a need to develop a base of research that supports the successful outcomes of the youth and community development approach. Although there are numerous programs operating and anecdotal stories that indicate successes, there needs to be stronger evidence of successful outcomes.

CONCLUSION

Youth development is a positive approach for African American youth because it encourages and respects their ideas and provides opportunities for them to be involved. The importance of positive adults within the lives of urban teens is crucial to the personal development of each youth, but ultimately for the community as a whole.

For too long, society has focused on the negative contributions of the few and ignored those who were doing positive things. Youth must be encouraged to be participant citizens in order to develop into participant citizen adults.

> *I am more convinced than ever of the importance of reinventing community, both within our schools and within our neighborhoods. This sense of place, of belonging, is a crucial building block for the healthy development of children and adolescents. And it is especially crucial for young people who are growing up in disadvantaged circumstances–the young people who face the most serious obstacles on the pathway to adulthood.*

–James P. Comer, Co-Chair, Task Force on Youth Development and
Community Programs

REFERENCES

Bloom, M. (1990). The psychosocial constructs of social competency. In T. P. Gullotta, G. R. Adams, and R. Montemeyor (Eds.). *Developing social competency in adolescence.* Newbury Park, CA: Sage Publications, (11-427).

Carnegie Council on Adolescent Development. (1992). *A matter of time: Risk and opportunities in the non-school hours.* Washington, D.C.: Author.

Dunkle, M. (1997). *Steer, row, or abandon ship: Re-thinking the federal role for children, youth, and families.* The Institute for Educational Leadership, The Policy Exchange, Special Report #8, 4.

Freedman, M. (1992). *The kindness of strangers.* Philadelphia, PA: Public Private Ventures.

Gambone, M. A. (1997). *Launching a resident driven initiative–Community change for youth development (CCYD) from Site Implementation to Early Implementation.* Philadelphia, PA: Public/Private Ventures.

Gullotta, T. P. (1990). Preface. In T. P. Gullotta, G. R. Adams, and R. Montemeyor (Eds.). *Developing social competency in adolescence.* Newbury Park, CA: Sage Publications, 7-8.

Johnson, B.R., Jeng, S. J., DeLi, S., and Larson, D. (2000). Black youth crises: The church as an agency of local social control, *Journal of Youth and Adolescence*, Vol. 25, No.4, 479-98.

Markstrom, C. A. (1999). Religious involvement and adolescent psychological development. *Journal of Adolescence*, 22, 205-225.

Meister, G. R. (1999). *The after-school initiative: The first five years* (Report); Hartford, CT: Hartford Foundation for Public Giving.

National Urban League, Education and Youth Development Program, Retrieved March 8, 2001 from the World Wide Web (*http://cgi.nul.org*).

Pittman, K., Irby, M., and Ferber, T. (2000). Unfinished business: Further reflections on a decade of promoting youth development. In *Youth development: Issues, challenges, and directions*, Philadelphia, PA: Public/Private Ventures.

Quinn, J. (1995). Positive effects of participation in youth organizations. In M. Rutter (Ed.). *Psychological disturbances in young people: Challenges for prevention.* New York: Cambridge University Press.

Roehlkepartain, E. C. and Benson, P. L. (1996). *Healthy communities healthy youth: A national initiative of Search Institute to unite communities for children and adolescents.* Minneapolis, MN: Search Institute.

Saito, R. N., Benson, P. L., Blythe, D. A., and Sharma, A. R. (1995). *Plans to grow: Perspectives on youth development opportunities for seven to fourteen year old Minnesota youth.* Minneapolis, MN: Search Institute.

Scales, P. and Leffer, N. (1999). *Developmental assets: A synthesis of the scientific research on adolescent development.* Minneapolis, MN: Search Institute.

Strive Media Institute. Retrieved March 15, 2001 from the World Wide Web (*www.strivemediainstitute.org*).

Synder, H. N. and Sickmund, M. (1999). *Juvenile offenders and victims: 1999 national report.* Washington, D.C.: Office of Juvenile Justice and Delinquency Prevention, U.S. Department of Justice.

The College Board. (1999). *Reaching the top. A report of the National Task Force on Minority High Achievement*, College Entrance Examination Board.

Walker, G. (2000). Introduction and overview. In *Youth development: Issues, challenges, and directions.* Philadelphia, PA: Public Private Ventures.

University of Wisconsin-Milwaukee, Youth Development Certificate Program. Retrieved February 20, 2001 from the World Wide Web (*www.uwm.edu/UniversityOutreach/catalog/CYCLC/youthdevel.shtml*).

The Plight
of the African American Student:
A Result of a Changing
School Environment

Sabra R. Smith, MA, EdD

SUMMARY. Educational problems of African American students are examined in the context of why young, successful early elementary school students are suddenly struggling in the late elementary and middle school years. Educators need to explore the educational environment, teacher attitudes and expectations, student empowerment, and the appropriateness of the curriculum. *[Article copies available for a fee from The Haworth Document Delivery Service: 1-800-HAWORTH. E-mail address: <getinfo@haworthpressinc.com> Website: <http://www.HaworthPress.com> © 2002 by The Haworth Press, Inc. All rights reserved.]*

KEYWORDS. Education, curriculum, African American, student empowerment

INTRODUCTION

Like other young children, African American children enter school with an immense level of excitement and fortitude–expressive, enthusi-

---

Sabra R. Smith is affiliated with the Institute of Scholar Training and Academic Tutorial (S.T.A.T) and is the owner and director of Angel Babies Childcare.

[Haworth co-indexing entry note]: "The Plight of the African American Student: A Result of a Changing School Environment." Smith, Sabra R. Co-published simultaneously in *Journal of Health & Social Policy* (The Haworth Press, Inc.) Vol. 15, No. 2, 2002, pp. 25-33; and: *African-American Adolescents in the Urban Community: Social Services Policy and Practice Interventions* (ed: Judith L. Rozie-Battle) The Haworth Press, Inc., 2002, pp. 25-33. Single or multiple copies of this article are available for a fee from The Haworth Document Delivery Service [1-800-HAWORTH, 9:00 a.m. - 5:00 p.m. (EST). E-mail address: getinfo@haworthpressinc.com].

astic, and creative. By the time they turn nine years old, however, the age at which most children enter the fourth grade, the level of energy that so propelled their spirited minds and bodies during the early childhood years diminishes. Apathetic, less focused on schooling, and an increased interest in sports, peers, and being cool, are some of the characteristics that African American children begin to display, particularly African American males (Kunjufu, 1985; Majors and Mancini-Billson, 1992). What happens in the early elementary grades that contributes to the plummeting academic performance of African American children? Why are so many of our children eager to learn and participate as students of Head Start and kindergarten, only to become unresponsive and disinterested in school by the fourth grade?

Some have referred to this phenomenon as the "Fourth Grade Failure Syndrome" (Kunjufu, 1985). Others have identified nine as the age at which most children begin to break away from their parents' identity and start to seek the own identities or "winning formulas" (Kiyosaki, 2001). Consequently, children who feel academically successful during this time of self-discovery, identify school as part of their winning formula. Those who fail to factor academia into the winning equation begin to include such things as playing sports, fostering relationships with peers, and being cool, things at which they are successful. It is during this time that African American children experience a loss of enthusiasm and trust in their schools and teachers.

TRANSFORMATION OF THE SCHOOL ENVIRONMENT

The early school years are comprised of classrooms that are both welcoming and inviting, with teachers who encourage self-expression and creativity. In this environment, young students are allowed to talk freely, imaginatively, and enthusiastically expressing their joys and sorrows, strengths, and weaknesses. They are also allowed to play with blocks and toys, to giggle, to walk around the classroom, and to collaboratively interact with other students. This environment revolves about the learning experiences of the child while teachers serve as guiding and nurturing supports.

As students advance in age and grade level, however, this familiar environment transforms from one that is student-centered to one that is teacher-centered. The heuristic and empowering climate of the early school years is changed to a climate of restricted behavior, competitiveness, and expected perfection in the area of verbal-linguistics. Teachers begin to take on dominant roles and make deposits of information into students as though they were empty receptacles waiting to be filled. Students are expected to receive, file, and store information, with an ability to accurately retrieve and regurgitate it upon request (Freire, 1970). Although people learn by making mistakes, beyond the very early years of schooling, the current school system punishes students for making too many mistakes. Yet, students who do not do well in school, usually do not have strong verbal-linguistic abilities, and do not learn by sitting still, listening, and taking notes. It is this abrupt transformation in the learning environment of the traditional American school that contributes to a distressed transition from the early years of schooling to the late primary school years for African American children, children who by nature are expressive, collaborative, and physical learners. The current school system is not designed to accommodate the learning styles of all children. According to Kiyosaki (2001), "The school system is not really a system of education as much as a system of elimination. . . . It is a system that is failing, not the kids."

THE TRADITIONAL SCHOOL SYSTEM

As African American children develop, they become aware of inequalities that exist within American society (Polite, 1999). They begin to identify inequalities within the school system, and soon establish views of the traditional American school as a hostile environment (Goggins, 1996). Although 40% of urban, public schools are populated by minority students, over 80% of urban school teachers are typically White, female, and about 40 years of age (Chase, 1998; Goggins, 1996; Los Angeles Times, 1998). In order to reach African American students, teachers must be able to identify with them through their language, their culture and their background. School curricula must be culturally relevant, and broadly based so as to empower students from diverse backgrounds and intelligence levels. Teachers must also develop higher expectations of young African American children through an acquired knowledge of their lives both inside and outside of the classroom. As it stands, the current school system teaches to one intelligence, the verbal-linguistic intelligence, and because they do not understand them, mainstream teachers have low expectations of African American students.

Curriculum

Through the pronounced use of English as a language form, superior to cultural languages like Spanish and Ebonics, and the subtleties of racism and structural inequalities embedded within school practices, school becomes an unwelcoming place to the African American student (Delpit, 1995; Tatum, 1997). While it is known that language is a powerful transmitter of culture and difference (Delpit, 1995; Hale-Benson, 1986; Kunjufu, 1989), school curricula legitimates dominant culture values by failing to include the language and backgrounds of subordinate groups like people of color, women, and the working class (Aronowitz and Giroux, 1985).

Domination is readily visible in American schools and is tightly woven into the fabric of classroom curriculum (Darder, 1991; Giroux, 1981). A study conducted on the content of books used in public schools found social studies books to be overly populated with themes that support dominant culture values (Anyon, 1980). An 80% to 20% ratio was found in a separate study that was intended to identify the percentage of mainstream to non-mainstream representation in literary selections (King, 1995). Biased curriculums, undiversified faculties and the ethos of traditional American schools leave African American students with feelings of detachment and discouragement (Hanssen, 1998; Welch and Hodges, 1997). This internalized rejection contributes to an underlying indifference towards school. The problem between school curriculum and the African American student lies in the cultural relationship between traditional schooling and the student (Irvine, 1991).

School Culture

Cognition is related to culture. Students who share a school's culture and behavior are more successful (Madhubuti and Madhubuti, 1994; Kunjufu, 1989). Original cognitive studies identify two styles of information processing and learning, the analytical style and the relational style (Cohen, 1969). Amongst several traits, analytical thinkers are stimulus centered, have long attention spans, and develop relationships that tend to be static and descriptive. Relational thinkers are self-centered, have short attention and concentration spans, and develop relationships that tend to be functional and inferential (Hillard, 1976). Traditional American curriculum is based on an analytical approach to cognition, while African American students are generally relational type thinkers.

In addition to a difference in learning style, there are several intelligences that African American students possess other than verbal-linguistic, the intellectual standard of the traditional school system. The difference between the culture that African American students bring to school and the standard culture of the school poses a problem for them. Consequently, the dissonance that African American students experience between demonstrated effort and emanated success contributes to a poor academic performance and an uncertainty of intellectual ability. When children experience academic failure, as measured by the traditional school standard, they begin to embrace ideas like, "I'm not smart" and "I'm stupid." It is at this time that African American children start to develop low self-esteem and poor attitudes about school. These children, the same children who entered school with an immense level of excitement and fortitude–expressive, enthusiastic, and creative, now hate school.

THE STRUGGLING AFRICAN AMERICAN STUDENT

Studies have confirmed that discrimination and repeated academic failure on the part of the African American student have led to a historical association between academic success and acting White (Ogbu, 1986; Singham, 1998; Tatum, 1997). Young African American students are conditioned to believe that academic success is something that is not a part of their culture. Many of them believe that if they try to conform to the expectations of White-dominated schools, they will be accused of "acting White" by their peers, and will experience feelings of losing sight of their own culture (Majors and Mancini-Billson, 1992). According to Singham, "The attempt by an individual Black to achieve academic success is seen as a betrayal because it would involve eventually conforming to the norms of White behavior and attitudes" (Singham, 1998, p. 11).

The African American Male

The socialization of the African American male into the peer group occurs at a very early age. Instead of a motivation towards academics, the African American male is motivated to be accepted by his peers and to demonstrate a "cool" demeanor. For many years, acting cool has served to enhance the black male's ability to withstand the harsh effects of racism and social oppression (Majors and Billson, 1992). Taking on a "cool" personality helps the Black male to achieve balance by allowing him to portray a sense of pride and dignity about himself. To him, the peer group serves as a sense of security and social support while society fosters a world of isolationism, racism, anxiety, and distress. Influenced by the older boys of the group, the young Black male becomes an ex-officio member when he: learns to walk distinctively (pimping); becomes athletically inclined; begins sexual explorations or can talk about his sexual prowess; becomes street-wise; earns an income for special needs or to assist his family; and learns to play the dozens, a cultural game of verbal insults requiring participants to suppress their emotions while at the same time developing rhythmic insults to revile back to their opponent (Hale-Benson, 1986). The young, African American male is "cool" when he is able to demonstrate these characteristics at any given time.

Understanding the African American Student

Oftentimes, teachers misinterpret the words and actions of African American students. The African American student's apparent defiance toward academia is a way of not "acting White." Taught in the classrooms of White, female teachers, African American males in particular, view academia as effeminate and academic success as something that is not culturally relevant. When teachers begin to understand these underlying assumptions, they will be able to identify with the African American student. It is when teachers are able to identify with the student, that they are able to engage them in the learning process rather than involve them in a continuous process of teacher-directed instruction, a form that African American students are not culturally accustomed to and often rebel against. Teachers empower students when they serve as active participants in the development of the student's unique voice within the school environment (Freire, 1970).

Student Empowerment

By engaging students in culturally relevant curriculums, teachers empower them to identify with their unique voice (Darder, 1991; Freire, 1970; McLaren, 1988). According to Delpit (1985), this voice is the linguistic form that students bring to school with them and is intimately tied to their home environment, family, and personal identity. "Culturally relevant teaching uses student culture in order to maintain it and to transcend the negative effects of the dominant culture" (Ladson-Billings, 1994). Ladson-Billings explains that the purpose of this type of teaching is to develop a cultural personality, which allows African American students the ability to choose academia while still allowing them to identify with their own culture.

Teachers must also empower students by incorporating methods into their curriculums that will address multiple intelligences. Students have intelligences that if tapped into, will increase their self-esteem and empower them to become academically successful.

TEACHER EXPECTATIONS OF AFRICAN AMERICAN STUDENTS

While the school's curriculum and environment are out of sync with the learning styles and cultural backgrounds of African American students, the lack of understanding between students and teachers often leads to stereotyping. A study used to randomly survey teachers and their feelings about Black students going on to college received negative replies from 60% of its respondents. According to this report, "teachers are susceptible to internalizing and projecting negative stereotypes and myths unfairly used to describe African American males" (Garibaldi, 1992). Teachers often allow their perception of a student to interfere with their ability to effectively teach them. When teachers have a misunderstanding of a student's potential, they tend to "underteach" the student despite the pedagogical practice (Delpit, 1985). When students are perceived as smart, they perform exceptionally (Kiyosaki, 2001).

IMPLICATIONS AND RECOMMENDATIONS

Young, African American children, as do most other children, enter school innately enthused about learning. Ironically, these same children by the time that they are nine-years-old begin to demonstrate a desire to leave school, to separate from dominant culture values and practices, and to become accepted by their peers. Disengaging from academics both mentally and physically, these students who were creatively engaged in learning and outspoken in the preschool and kindergarten environments, begin to lash out in the classroom.

Changes in the climate of the academic classroom, traditional American school curricula and culture, misunderstandings of the African American student, and low teacher expectations have been presented as factors, which contribute to the young, African American's plummeting performance and disinterest in school. As indicated by the original studies of Cohen (1969) and Hillard (1976), the learning styles of students vary by culture. African American students, generally relational type thinkers, tend to be less analytically minded than their mainstream counterparts.

An early indication of the African American student's propensity to reject academia is seen in the level of success during the primary school years, after kindergarten. If African American students experience repeated failure, there is a strong possibility that their academic performance will plummet, as well as their levels of self-esteem. Teachers must include practices that will support the learning styles of all students. Whether they are visual learners or kinesthetic learners, school curricula should be designed to draw the maximum amount of success from the maximum amount of students. Early experiences of academic success can circumvent a diversion from schooling.

The African American student must also be socialized to believe that being Black and smart is acceptable. Embedded within the curriculum there must be concepts, ideas, and practices that identify with the language and background of African American people. Schools must empower students both mainstream and non-mainstream. Through a positive experience of schooling, young African American children will be able to make a favorable transition from the early years of kindergarten to the primary grades and into the intermediate, secondary, and higher learning school years. The only way to redirect a downward spiral of the academic performance of the African American student is to restructure traditional school curriculum and its implementation. All students must be able to identify with the curriculum and practice of school, which helps to shape a perception of themselves that is likely to follow them the rest of their lives. Schools must be socialized to accept and act upon the differences that each student brings with them. A body is only as strong as its weakest member. Until the system, as a whole, works to strengthen and empower its subordinate groups, it will always remain plagued with underachievement. In the words of Booker T. Washington:

> *There is no defense or security for any of us except in the highest intelligence and development of all.*

–Booker T. Washington
September 18, 1895

REFERENCES

Anyon, J. (1980). Social class and the hidden curriculum of work. *Journal of Education*, 162,121-126.

Aronowitz, S., and Giroux, H. (1985). *Education under siege*. New York: Bergin and Garvey.

Chase, B. (1998). Wanted: Minority teachers desperately seeking diverse and excellent educators. *The Washington Post, January 11th*, C5.

Cohen, R. (1969). Conceptual styles, culture conflict and nonverbal tests of intelligence. *American Anthropologist*, 71,828-56.

Darder, A. (1991). *Culture and power in the classroom.* Westport, CT: Bergin and Garvey.

Delpit, L. (1995). *Other people's children: Cultural conflict in the classroom.* New York: The New Press.

Freire, P. (1970). *Pedagogy of the oppressed.* New York: Continuum.

Garibaldi, A. M. (1992). Educating and motivating African American males to succeed. *Journal of Negro Education,* 61(1).

Giroux, H. (1981). *Ideology, culture, and the process of schooling.* Philadelphia: Temple University Press.

Goggins, L. II. (1996). *African centered rites of passage and education.* Illinois: African American Images.

Hale-Benson, J. (1986). *Black children: Their roots, culture, and learning styles.* Baltimore: Johns Hopkins University Press.

Hanssen, E. (1998). A White teacher reflects on institutional racism. *Phi Delta Kappa,* May, 79(9).

Hillard, A. (1976). *Alternatives to IQ testing: An approach to the identification of gifted minority children.* Final report to the California State Department of Education.

Irvine, J. J. (1991). *Black students and school failure.* New York: Praeger.

King, G. P. (1995). *Researching biases in curriculum and instructional content.* 34-03. University of Houston.

Kiyosaki, R. T. (2001). *Rich kid smart kid: Giving your child a financial head start.* New York: Warner Books.

Kunjufu, J. (1985). *Countering the conspiracy to destroy black boys.* IL: African American Images.

Kunjufu, J. (1989). *Critical issues in educating African American youth.* IL: African American Images.

Ladson-Billings, G. (1994). *The dreamkeepers: Successful teachers of African American children.* San Francisco: Jossey-Bass.

Los Angeles Times. (1998). Public education: California's perilous slide–Little training, poor oversight. *Los Angeles Times,* May 19.

Madhubuti, H., and Madhubuti, S. (1994). *African-centered education: Its value, importance and necessity in the development of black children.* Chicago: Third World Press.

Majors, R., and Mancini-Billson, J. (1992). *Cool pose: The dilemmas of black manhood in American.* New York: Touchstone Simon and Schuster Inc.

McLaren, P. (1988). *Life in schools: An introduction to critical pedagogy in the foundations of education.* New York: Longman.

Ogbu, J. U. (1986). The consequences of the American caste system. In U. Neisser (Ed.), *The school achievement of minority children: New perspectives.* Hillsdale, NJ: Lawrence Erlbaum Associates.

Polite, V. C. and Davis, J. E. (Eds.) (1999). *African American males in school and society: Practices and policies for effective education.* New York: Teachers College Press.

Singham, M. (1998). The canary in the mine: The achievement gap between black and white students. *Phi Delta Kappan,* September.

Tatum, B. D. (1997). *Why are all the black kids sitting together in the cafeteria and other conversations about race.* New York: Basic Books.

Welch, O. M., and Hodges, C. R. (1997). *Standing outside on the inside.* Albany: State University of New York Press.

Health Concerns
for African American Youth

Stanley F. Battle, MSW, MPH, PhD

SUMMARY. African American youth today face many challenges that can result in poor decisions and lead to high risk behavior. This nation has experienced a decrease in the number of teen pregnancies, but among African American youth the rates are still too high. African American youth also struggle with alcohol and drug addiction and limited access to health care. In short, there are many challenges to providing appropriate health care to our youth. *[Article copies available for a fee from The Haworth Document Delivery Service: 1-800-HAWORTH. E-mail address: <getinfo@haworthpressinc.com> Website: <http://www.HaworthPress.com> © 2002 by The Haworth Press, Inc. All rights reserved.]*

KEYWORDS. Health, African American youth, teen pregnancy, substance abuse

INTRODUCTION

As a result of the astounding scientific and medical achievements of the twentieth century, we know a fuller measure of health is within reach for all children in the United States. Yet, despite the overall achievements in health status, the burden of poor health all too often falls more heavily on some population groups than on others. The fact

---

Stanley F. Battle is Vice Chancellor of Student and Multicultural Affairs at the University of Wisconsin-Milwaukee.

[Haworth co-indexing entry note]: "Health Concerns for African American Youth." Battle, Stanley F. Co-published simultaneously in *Journal of Health & Social Policy* (The Haworth Press, Inc.) Vol. 15, No. 2, 2002, pp. 35-44; and: *African-American Adolescents in the Urban Community: Social Services Policy and Practice Interventions* (ed: Judith L. Rozie-Battle) The Haworth Press, Inc., 2002, pp. 35-44. Single or multiple copies of this article are available for a fee from The Haworth Document Delivery Service [1-800-HAWORTH, 9:00 a.m. - 5:00 p.m. (EST). E-mail address: getinfo@haworthpressinc.com].

that this "gap" in health status occurs more frequently among people with low income and racial/ethnic "minority" groups has been documented nationally. These groups are identified as African American, Hispanic/Latino, and to a lesser degree, Asian and Pacific Islanders. The health and development of children is a major challenge for the United States. Health care gaps experienced by these multi-ethnic groups include consistently higher mortality and poorer overall health–as measured by infant mortality rates and disability levels. The gap involves disparities in health-related information and resources as well.

The challenge of ensuring good health for all residents is of critical importance in multi-ethnic communities because population growth has shifted and these groups must provide leadership for the country. Minority populations are now majority populations in many areas. Strategies to improve health must be based on the fullest possible knowledge of influences on health and illness for particular population groups. But more often than not, strategies to improve the health of multi-ethnic groups are transplanted or adapted from interventions and research based on middle-income Whites.

Unfortunately, differences in culture, race, and language are all too often treated as a series of obstacles, which must be overcome in providing health care services.

Reaching the goal of equitable health status for all multi-ethnic children will be the most important public health achievement of our time. Good health and well-being are the greatest legacies we can leave our children and future generations (Adams, 1993).

TEEN PREGNANCIES

The numbers are familiar, each year more than one million American teenagers become pregnant. Of those, one half million give birth. Most of these adolescents are unmarried, and many are not ready for the responsibilities and demands of parenthood. However, there is some cause to be hopeful. In a recent study done by the Annie E. Casey Foundation, the findings showed that "since 1991, the percentages of American teenagers getting pregnant, giving birth, or having abortions have all fallen. Teen pregnancies have declined 14 percent since 1990, reaching the lowest annual rate in more than 20 years. These declines occurred in every state and the District of Columbia and across all racial groups."

ales under the age of 20 have rates of infection with chlamydia
homatis that are 2-3 times higher than females over 20. In cases
rrhea, nationally, teens represent 25% of reported cases.

SUBSTANCE ABUSE

g the 1980s, crack cocaine use by African Americans grew so
cally that most African American communities were in their
lecade of a crack cocaine epidemic by the 1990s. The marketing
y addictive, low-cost "crack" has changed the very fabric of ur-
ican American life. Increased crime, prostitution, and gang vio-
s resulted in a "War on Drugs," which has more often appeared
war on addicts. In the United States, substance abuse has been
d as an African American problem (Walker-Jones and Ford,

ance abuse–abuse of alcohol, prescription, or illicit drugs–is a
ecognized public health problem in the United States. Alco-
ed disorders are the more prevalent of the two types. However,
dependencies often co-exist. A sharp upswing in adolescent
began in the mid-70s, preceded by a marked increase of usage
ge students about 10 years earlier. Drugs had always been avail-
never were they used in such high quantity by such young peo-
er had use been socially acceptable nor the myth of harmlessness
y believed. Previously, illicit drug use in our culture was typi-
ondition of people in economic or personal distress. The heroin
the ghetto was the prototype. The drugs abused prior to 1960
st often the opiates well-known for their ability to relieve pain.
cal adolescent drug abuser in the 1990s does not fit the picture
40 drug abuser. His and her socioeconomic status and drug
ave changed markedly.
lerable confusion exists among adults, physicians, and others
about the relationship of juvenile drinking and drug abuse.
ve been quick to point out that adult society consumes large
of alcohol in various forms, and adolescents see it as more dan-
an their drug of choice, marijuana. Adults, who say that they
hat their child uses no drugs, although well aware of their alco-
heed to develop a better understanding of the relationship be-
gs and alcohol. Any person who consumes enough alcohol on
s to cause even occasional problems with driving or social situ-
s a drug problem (Walker-Jones and Ford, 1998).

Researchers cite two main reasons for the overall drop in both pregnancy and birth rates: Fewer teens are having sex, and among those who
are, more are using contraceptives. In a special analysis of the falling
pregnancy and birth rates, Patricia Donovan of the Alan Guttmacher Institute (AGI) noted that teens are placing a greater emphasis on delaying
sexual activity, holding to more responsible attitudes among teenagers
about casual sex and out-of wedlock childbearing, showing heightened
fear of sexually transmitted diseases–especially AIDS, and using
long-lasting contraceptive methods, such as the implant (Norplant) and
the injectable (Depo-Provera) options. The researchers also point out
the pregnancy rates decline in an economic boom, when teens have
better job prospects and are not as hopelessly trapped on the bottom of
the socioeconomic ladder.

As reported in *When Teens Have Sex: Issues and Trends* issued by the
Annie E. Casey Foundation (1998), demographic trends confirm that the
recent good news may be short-lived. "As the children of the 'baby
boomlet' swell the ranks of American teenagers over the next few years,"
the Foundation reports, "the absolute number of babies born to teenagers
is likely to increase even if the birth rate remains constant."

National data does not reflect urban conditions. In Milwaukee, Wisconsin teenage births accounted for almost twice as many (20.8 percent)
of the total births as they did for the state of Wisconsin (10.7 percent). In
1997, City of Milwaukee teen births accounted for 92 percent and 31.6
percent of all teen births in Milwaukee County and the state of Wisconsin, respectively. During the same year, well over half of all teen births
were to Blacks. Further reviews of the data reveal a downward trend but
they are still higher than the national rate. In short, Black Milwaukee is
home to a disproportionately high number of Wisconsin's teenage
mother and fathers (Wisconsin Department of Health, 1998).

One of the concerns is the elevated rate of teen pregnancies in urban
communities. By utilizing contraceptions, pregnancies can be prevented, as well as the spread of AIDS.

Contrary to the positive changes in communicable diseases, rates of
AIDS in Milwaukee increased by 32% between 1990 and 1997. This
type of data reveals ongoing challenges to the health care delivery systems and reinforces the fact that socioeconomic and demographic shifts
within and around a community requires diligent disease monitoring.
Therefore, health professionals must recognize successful efforts
(Washington, 2000).

Out of seven persons contracting HIV daily, three of those are African-Americans in this country. Even though, there has been a decline in

HIV/AIDS death rates due to new therapies, AIDS is the number one killer of African American males between the ages of 25 and 44 years and is the second leading cause of death among African American women of the same age group (U.S. Department of Health and Human Services, 1999).

It is also known that condom use is lower and teen pregnancy higher in occurrence in African American teens (Jemmott, 1992). This places African American teens at higher risk for HIV/AIDS. African American teens make up 15% of the American adolescent population, but in some cities account for 38% of the AIDS cases among this group (New York City Department of Health, 1994). Gonorrhea remains the most common sexually transmitted disease (STD) among adolescents, nationwide (Judson, 1990).

Despite the decreases in teenage pregnancy, AIDS continues to be a significant challenge in African American communities.

To fully understand the impact of this problem on Black Milwaukee, it is useful to step back and look at the national stage, where public officials, community groups, and ordinary citizens are taking different approaches to meeting the special needs of teenage parents and their children. In the past, most of the effort was aimed at stigmatizing and isolating teens under the guise of teen pregnancy prevention programs. But Dorothy Stoneman, executive director of YouthBuild U.S.A., has another perspective that provides Black Milwaukee with an excellent starting point:

> The government's perspective is the short term. You have a bad situation and you provide short-term intervention, getting someone out of alienation into the mainstream in a way that is basically obedient. But you need a community in which people can grow up, that has values, aspirations, and support systems. Instead, we have communities in which institutions are not working, and so the people who survive are the exceptions. It is not that a few people have deficits and therefore they can't make it and they need productive programs. It is that most of the people are not getting what they need from the community. Therefore, we need to rebuild communities in which people can grow up in a healthy context.

SEXUALLY TRANSMITTED DISEASES (STDs)

The most common STDs are chlamydia, trichomoniasis, gonorrhea and syphilis. Chlamydia–the most common–is a bacteria that lives in cells. Females can develop pelvic inflammatory disease, which can lead to serious complications and infertility. Trich[...] organism found in 3-40% of the male partners[...] orrhea is generally easier to detect in males th[...] usually appear within 3 to 5 days after sexua[...] person. About 80% of infected females show[...] ilis is less common but more dangerous than g[...] occur about 3-4 weeks after contact, as early a[...] as long as 3 months after contact.

Sexually transmitted diseases have becom[...] adolescents and college students. There are m[...] mitted diseases which account annually for i[...] lion U.S. teenagers (Walker-Jones and Ford,[...]

Healthy People 2000, estimated that there [...] of STDs reported in the United States. A repo[...] within the population of 15-29 year-olds of th[...] of Health and Human Services, 1996). Sexual[...] ten progress more rapidly in adolescents, sh[...] orrhea, chlamydia, and syphilis. It is impor[...] STDs relate to each other. For example, trich[...] the development of genital warts (herpes). [...] spread and unpleasant STD, caused by a virus[...] painful genital sores, blisters, pain, and sev[...] ver, muscle aches, and other general symp[...] cently, studies suggest that STDs such [...] eruptions or sores–may facilitate the transm[...] Important during adolescent years is the [...] While lice are usually transmitted by sexual[...] transmitted by contaminated clothes or bedd[...] be aware that the presence of one or more se[...] greatly increases your likelihood of contrac[...]

African American teens show the greatest[...] justed rates in Black males being 15 times hi[...] terparts. In addition, when compared to Whit[...] females show increased risk of death due t[...] ease (PID) and syphilis (Wisconsin Depart[...] Services, 1990).

In the United States, about half the teena[...] sexually active. Because they are initiating [...] agers are at increasingly high risk for acq[...] diseases. Each year teenagers represent app[...] national STD cases (Centers for Disease C[...]

In 1998, the Monitoring the Future (MTF) Study asked a nationally representative sample of nearly 50,000 secondary school students in public and private schools to describe their drug use patterns through self-administered questionnaires. Surveying seniors annually since 1975, the study expanded in 1991 to include 8th and 10th graders. By design, MTF excludes dropouts and institutionalized, homeless, and runaway youth.

In 1998, 54% of all seniors said they had at least tried illicit drugs. Marijuana was by far the most commonly used illicit drug: In 1998, 49% of high school seniors said they had tried marijuana. About half of those who said they had used marijuana (or 25% of all seniors) said they had not used any other illicit drug. About 3 in 10 seniors (29%) (or slightly more than half of seniors who used illicit drugs) had used an illicit drug other than marijuana (Synder and Sickmund, 1999).

Moreover, 4 in 5 high school seniors said they had tried alcohol at least once; half said they had used it in the previous month. Even among 8th graders, the use of alcohol was high: one-half had tried alcohol, and almost one-quarter had used it in the month prior to the survey (Synder and Sickmund, 1999).

Perhaps of greater concern are the juveniles who indicated heavy drinking (defined as five or more drinks in a row) in the preceding 2 weeks: 31% of seniors, 24% of 10th graders, and 14% of 8th graders reported this behavior.

According to the Centers for Disease Control and Prevention's 1997 Youth Risk Behavior Surveillance Survey, 6% of high school students said they had had at least one drink of alcohol on school property in the past month. Similarly, 7% said they had used marijuana on school property during the same time period (Synder and Sickmund, 1999).

The data should raise concern on the part of health and social service providers, as well as policy makers. Yet, these numbers exclude the findings of use by some of the most disenfranchised youth. The dropouts, runaways, and others not included will most likely provide a more bleak picture than the young people surveyed, who are still involved with the educational system.

HEALTH INSURANCE

The proportion of children in this nation covered by private health insurance has decreased in recent years, to 66% of all children in 1996. During the preceding ten years before 1996, the proportion of children receiving public health insurance, i.e., Medicaid had grown from 19% to 25%. Hispanic children are less likely to have health insurance than non-Hispanic, White or African-American children. The rate of child health coverage varies little by age, but younger children (birth to 5 years) are more likely than older children to have public (rather than private) health insurance. More than half of the poor children use public rather than private health insurance, and nearly twice as many poor children are uninsured compared to near-poor children (Willis, 2000).

Assessments for the insured and uninsured populations, repeatedly support that Wisconsin is one of this nation's leading states in health insurance coverage for its citizens. The Medical Expenditure Panel Survey (MEPS) of 1996 supports that African-Americans and Hispanics are more likely than Whites to be uninsured. African-Americans are more likely to be publicly insured, and whites are more likely to have private coverage.

The impact that managed care organizations (with the fundamental premise to contain costs) have on under served ethnic groups continues to be studied. Some health policy experts have concluded that the utilization review process in managed care organizations will not abate accessibility for minorities to health care because they have more severe conditions that require more intensive therapy. They assert that disadvantaged groups are in greater need of health care. Ironically though, others believe that the managed care system, as an alternative care plan to the fee for service, essentially sustains access barriers to health care for minorities and the poor. State and federal health policy persons must continue to examine how race and ethnicity impact the amount and quality of health care for patients (Willis, 2000).

When federal researchers analyzed Medicaid discharges by hospital ownership and degree of penetration of managed care organizations, they showed that public hospitals in central cities experienced the greatest loss of market shares, regardless of the increased uninsured population throughout this nation.

With a $2 trillion budget and a surplus projected over the next 10 years, a booming economy, and money from the tobacco settlement, we have an historic opportunity to invest in a better future for our children by investing in activities that promote their health and well-being (Children's Defense Fund, 2000).

Vermont ranks 1st in the nation with only 6.4 percent of children without health coverage, Arizona and Texas rank last with 25.9 percent and 25.3 percent (respectively) of children without health coverage (see Table 1) (Children's Defense Fund, 2000).

Researchers cite two main reasons for the overall drop in both pregnancy and birth rates: Fewer teens are having sex, and among those who
are, more are using contraceptives. In a special analysis of the falling
pregnancy and birth rates, Patricia Donovan of the Alan Guttmacher Institute (AGI) noted that teens are placing a greater emphasis on delaying
sexual activity, holding to more responsible attitudes among teenagers
about casual sex and out-of wedlock childbearing, showing heightened
fear of sexually transmitted diseases–especially AIDS, and using
long-lasting contraceptive methods, such as the implant (Norplant) and
the injectable (Depo-Provera) options. The researchers also point out
the pregnancy rates decline in an economic boom, when teens have
better job prospects and are not as hopelessly trapped on the bottom of
the socioeconomic ladder.

As reported in *When Teens Have Sex: Issues and Trends* issued by the
Annie E. Casey Foundation (1998), demographic trends confirm that the
recent good news may be short-lived. "As the children of the 'baby
boomlet' swell the ranks of American teenagers over the next few years,"
the Foundation reports, "the absolute number of babies born to teenagers
is likely to increase even if the birth rate remains constant."

National data does not reflect urban conditions. In Milwaukee, Wisconsin teenage births accounted for almost twice as many (20.8 percent)
of the total births as they did for the state of Wisconsin (10.7 percent). In
1997, City of Milwaukee teen births accounted for 92 percent and 31.6
percent of all teen births in Milwaukee County and the state of Wisconsin, respectively. During the same year, well over half of all teen births
were to Blacks. Further reviews of the data reveal a downward trend but
they are still higher than the national rate. In short, Black Milwaukee is
home to a disproportionately high number of Wisconsin's teenage
mother and fathers (Wisconsin Department of Health, 1998).

One of the concerns is the elevated rate of teen pregnancies in urban
communities. By utilizing contraceptions, pregnancies can be prevented, as well as the spread of AIDS.

Contrary to the positive changes in communicable diseases, rates of
AIDS in Milwaukee increased by 32% between 1990 and 1997. This
type of data reveals ongoing challenges to the health care delivery systems and reinforces the fact that socioeconomic and demographic shifts
within and around a community requires diligent disease monitoring.
Therefore, health professionals must recognize successful efforts
(Washington, 2000).

Out of seven persons contracting HIV daily, three of those are African-Americans in this country. Even though, there has been a decline in

HIV/AIDS death rates due to new therapies, AIDS is the number one killer of African American males between the ages of 25 and 44 years and is the second leading cause of death among African American women of the same age group (U.S. Department of Health and Human Services, 1999).

It is also known that condom use is lower and teen pregnancy higher in occurrence in African American teens (Jemmott, 1992). This places African American teens at higher risk for HIV/AIDS. African American teens make up 15% of the American adolescent population, but in some cities account for 38% of the AIDS cases among this group (New York City Department of Health, 1994). Gonorrhea remains the most common sexually transmitted disease (STD) among adolescents, nationwide (Judson, 1990).

Despite the decreases in teenage pregnancy, AIDS continues to be a significant challenge in African American communities.

To fully understand the impact of this problem on Black Milwaukee, it is useful to step back and look at the national stage, where public officials, community groups, and ordinary citizens are taking different approaches to meeting the special needs of teenage parents and their children. In the past, most of the effort was aimed at stigmatizing and isolating teens under the guise of teen pregnancy prevention programs. But Dorothy Stoneman, executive director of YouthBuild U.S.A., has another perspective that provides Black Milwaukee with an excellent starting point:

> The government's perspective is the short term. You have a bad situation and you provide short-term intervention, getting someone out of alienation into the mainstream in a way that is basically obedient. But you need a community in which people can grow up, that has values, aspirations, and support systems. Instead, we have communities in which institutions are not working, and so the people who survive are the exceptions. It is not that a few people have deficits and therefore they can't make it and they need productive programs. It is that most of the people are not getting what they need from the community. Therefore, we need to rebuild communities in which people can grow up in a healthy context.

SEXUALLY TRANSMITTED DISEASES (STDs)

The most common STDs are chlamydia, trichomoniasis, gonorrhea and syphilis. Chlamydia–the most common–is a bacteria that lives in cells. Females can develop pelvic inflammatory disease, which can lead to serious complications and infertility. Trichomoniasis is caused by an organism found in 3-40% of the male partners of infected women. Gonorrhea is generally easier to detect in males than in females. Symptoms usually appear within 3 to 5 days after sexual contact with an infected person. About 80% of infected females show no symptoms at all. Syphilis is less common but more dangerous than gonorrhea. Symptoms can occur about 3-4 weeks after contact, as early as 10 days after contact, or as long as 3 months after contact.

Sexually transmitted diseases have become more common among adolescents and college students. There are more than 30 sexually transmitted diseases which account annually for infections among 2.5 million U.S. teenagers (Walker-Jones and Ford, 1999).

Healthy People 2000, estimated that there have been 12 million cases of STDs reported in the United States. A reported 86% of the cases were within the population of 15-29 year-olds of the nation (U.S. Department of Health and Human Services, 1996). Sexually transmitted diseases often progress more rapidly in adolescents, showing higher rates of gonorrhea, chlamydia, and syphilis. It is important to recognize how the STDs relate to each other. For example, trichomoniasis may encourage the development of genital warts (herpes). Genital herpes is a widespread and unpleasant STD, caused by a virus. The first infection causes painful genital sores, blisters, pain, and severe itching. Headaches, fever, muscle aches, and other general symptoms can also occur. Recently, studies suggest that STDs such as herpes–involving skin eruptions or sores–may facilitate the transmission of the AIDS virus. Important during adolescent years is the recognition of pubic lice. While lice are usually transmitted by sexual intimacy, they can also be transmitted by contaminated clothes or bedding. All adolescents should be aware that the presence of one or more sexually transmitted diseases greatly increases your likelihood of contracting the AIDS virus.

African American teens show the greatest risk for STDs with age-adjusted rates in Black males being 15 times higher than their White counterparts. In addition, when compared to White females, Black adolescent females show increased risk of death due to pelvic inflammatory disease (PID) and syphilis (Wisconsin Department of Health and Social Services, 1990).

In the United States, about half the teenage population reports being sexually active. Because they are initiating sexual activity earlier, teenagers are at increasingly high risk for acquiring sexually transmitted diseases. Each year teenagers represent approximately 2 million of the national STD cases (Centers for Disease Control, 1989). Sexually active females under the age of 20 have rates of infection with chlamydia and trachomatis that are 2-3 times higher than females over 20. In cases of gonorrhea, nationally, teens represent 25% of reported cases.

SUBSTANCE ABUSE

During the 1980s, crack cocaine use by African Americans grew so dramatically that most African American communities were in their second decade of a crack cocaine epidemic by the 1990s. The marketing of highly addictive, low-cost "crack" has changed the very fabric of urban, African American life. Increased crime, prostitution, and gang violence has resulted in a "War on Drugs," which has more often appeared to be a war on addicts. In the United States, substance abuse has been portrayed as an African American problem (Walker-Jones and Ford, 1998).

Substance abuse–abuse of alcohol, prescription, or illicit drugs–is a widely recognized public health problem in the United States. Alcohol-related disorders are the more prevalent of the two types. However, the two dependencies often co-exist. A sharp upswing in adolescent drug use began in the mid-70s, preceded by a marked increase of usage by college students about 10 years earlier. Drugs had always been available, but never were they used in such high quantity by such young people. Never had use been socially acceptable nor the myth of harmlessness so widely believed. Previously, illicit drug use in our culture was typically a condition of people in economic or personal distress. The heroin addict of the ghetto was the prototype. The drugs abused prior to 1960 were most often the opiates well-known for their ability to relieve pain. The typical adolescent drug abuser in the 1990s does not fit the picture of the 1940 drug abuser. His and her socioeconomic status and drug choices have changed markedly.

Considerable confusion exists among adults, physicians, and others as well, about the relationship of juvenile drinking and drug abuse. Youth have been quick to point out that adult society consumes large amounts of alcohol in various forms, and adolescents see it as more dangerous than their drug of choice, marijuana. Adults, who say that they are glad that their child uses no drugs, although well aware of their alcohol use, need to develop a better understanding of the relationship between drugs and alcohol. Any person who consumes enough alcohol on weekends to cause even occasional problems with driving or social situations has a drug problem (Walker-Jones and Ford, 1998).

In 1998, the Monitoring the Future (MTF) Study asked a nationally representative sample of nearly 50,000 secondary school students in public and private schools to describe their drug use patterns through self-administered questionnaires. Surveying seniors annually since 1975, the study expanded in 1991 to include 8th and 10th graders. By design, MTF excludes dropouts and institutionalized, homeless, and runaway youth.

In 1998, 54% of all seniors said they had at least tried illicit drugs. Marijuana was by far the most commonly used illicit drug: In 1998, 49% of high school seniors said they had tried marijuana. About half of those who said they had used marijuana (or 25% of all seniors) said they had not used any other illicit drug. About 3 in 10 seniors (29%) (or slightly more than half of seniors who used illicit drugs) had used an illicit drug other than marijuana (Synder and Sickmund, 1999).

Moreover, 4 in 5 high school seniors said they had tried alcohol at least once; half said they had used it in the previous month. Even among 8th graders, the use of alcohol was high: one-half had tried alcohol, and almost one-quarter had used it in the month prior to the survey (Synder and Sickmund, 1999).

Perhaps of greater concern are the juveniles who indicated heavy drinking (defined as five or more drinks in a row) in the preceding 2 weeks: 31% of seniors, 24% of 10th graders, and 14% of 8th graders reported this behavior.

According to the Centers for Disease Control and Prevention's 1997 Youth Risk Behavior Surveillance Survey, 6% of high school students said they had had at least one drink of alcohol on school property in the past month. Similarly, 7% said they had used marijuana on school property during the same time period (Synder and Sickmund, 1999).

The data should raise concern on the part of health and social service providers, as well as policy makers. Yet, these numbers exclude the findings of use by some of the most disenfranchised youth. The dropouts, runaways, and others not included will most likely provide a more bleak picture than the young people surveyed, who are still involved with the educational system.

HEALTH INSURANCE

The proportion of children in this nation covered by private health insurance has decreased in recent years, to 66% of all children in 1996. During the preceding ten years before 1996, the proportion of children receiving public health insurance, i.e., Medicaid had grown from 19% to 25%. Hispanic children are less likely to have health insurance than non-Hispanic, White or African-American children. The rate of child health coverage varies little by age, but younger children (birth to 5 years) are more likely than older children to have public (rather than private) health insurance. More than half of the poor children use public rather than private health insurance, and nearly twice as many poor children are uninsured compared to near-poor children (Willis, 2000).

Assessments for the insured and uninsured populations, repeatedly support that Wisconsin is one of this nation's leading states in health insurance coverage for its citizens. The Medical Expenditure Panel Survey (MEPS) of 1996 supports that African-Americans and Hispanics are more likely than Whites to be uninsured. African-Americans are more likely to be publicly insured, and whites are more likely to have private coverage.

The impact that managed care organizations (with the fundamental premise to contain costs) have on under served ethnic groups continues to be studied. Some health policy experts have concluded that the utilization review process in managed care organizations will not abate accessibility for minorities to health care because they have more severe conditions that require more intensive therapy. They assert that disadvantaged groups are in greater need of health care. Ironically though, others believe that the managed care system, as an alternative care plan to the fee for service, essentially sustains access barriers to health care for minorities and the poor. State and federal health policy persons must continue to examine how race and ethnicity impact the amount and quality of health care for patients (Willis, 2000).

When federal researchers analyzed Medicaid discharges by hospital ownership and degree of penetration of managed care organizations, they showed that public hospitals in central cities experienced the greatest loss of market shares, regardless of the increased uninsured population throughout this nation.

With a $2 trillion budget and a surplus projected over the next 10 years, a booming economy, and money from the tobacco settlement, we have an historic opportunity to invest in a better future for our children by investing in activities that promote their health and well-being (Children's Defense Fund, 2000).

Vermont ranks 1st in the nation with only 6.4 percent of children without health coverage, Arizona and Texas rank last with 25.9 percent and 25.3 percent (respectively) of children without health coverage (see Table 1) (Children's Defense Fund, 2000).

TABLE 1. U.S. Assessment of Children Without Health Coverage

	Best States				Worst States		
Rank		Estimated number	Rate	Rank		Estimated number	Rate
1	Vermont	10,000	6.4%	51	Arizona	365,000	25.9%
2	Hawaii	22,000	6.8	50	Texas	1,565,000	25.3
3	Wisconsin	100,000	6.9	49	Arkansas	162,000	22.6
4	Rhode Island	19,000	7.5	48	Louisiana	284,000	21.4
5	Pennsylvania	255,000	8.3	47	Nevada	102,000	20.4
6	Nebraska	40,000	8.4	46	Mississippi	164,000	19.5
7	Minnesota	116,000	8.6	44	Florida	745,000	19.3
8	Massachusetts	138,000	8.9	44	California	1,881,000	19.3
9	Michigan	247,000	9.0	43	Oklahoma	179,000	18.5
10	South Dakota	20,000	9.1	42	South Carolina	193,000	18.2

PRINCIPLES FOR STRONG/HEALTH INSTITUTIONAL RELATIONSHIPS

Relationships must occur between multi-ethnic groups and health institutions at all levels, and certain guiding principles must drive these relationships:

- Extensive and early involvement in the strategic planning process of all health institutions is crucial.
- Persistent, honest, and open communications are essential.
- Continual development of credibility and trust.
- Willingness to admit and correct mistakes must pervade these processes.
- Collaborative approaches to problem solving need to always occur.
- Development of continuous and strong organizational leadership must be nurtured.
- Understanding of differences must be developed between how community leaders and health administrators think and act.

CONCLUSION

Who are we and how do we measure up to these principles? Our task is well-defined; it calls for *no more research*. The health needs of children are great, yet they are manageable. We must pursue a course of rational and practical action to release the inordinate burden of illness, productive years lost, and premature death. We are family and, therefore, special emphasis must be placed on recapturing the health of our children to free them from illness and behaviors that prevent them from learning, and falling into mediocracy, and rob them of their potential. The time to act is *now*.

REFERENCES

Adams, F. (1993). Health care in crisis. In S. Battle (Ed.). The state of Black Hartford. Hartford CT: Urban League of Greater Hartford: ITT Hartford Publisher, pp. 175-182.

The Annie E. Casey Foundation. (1998). When teens have sex: Issues and trends, KIDS Count, Special Report.

Centers for Disease Control. (1989). Division of STD/HIV prevention, annual report, Atlanta, GA.

Children in the states 2000. (2000). Children's Defense Fund 2000, Washington D.C.

U. S. Department of Health and Human Services. (1999). Closing the gap. The minority AIDS crisis. Office of Public Health and Science, Office of Minority Health, U. S. Department of Health and Human Services.

Jemmott, L. S. and J. B. Jemmott, 111. (1992). Increasing condom-use intentions among sexually active inner-city Black adolescent women: Effects of an AIDS prevention program. *Nursing Research*, 41, pp. 273-279.

Judson, F.N. (1990). Gonorrhea *Medical Clinics of North America*, Vol. 74 (6), pp. 1353-66.

Synder, H. N. and Sickmund, M. (1999). *Juvenile offenders and victims:1999 national report*. Washington, D.C.: Office of Juvenile Justice and Delinquency Prevention, U.S. Department of Justice.

U.S. Department of Health and Human Services. (1996). COC, Healthy people 2000: National health promotion and disease prevention objectives, Hyattsville, Maryland.

Walker-Jones, Y. and Ford, A. (1999). High risk behaviors: STDs and substance abuse. In Mason, A. and Bangs, R. (Eds.). The state of Black youth in Pittsburgh. Pittsburgh, PA: Urban League of Pittsburgh, pp. 252-261.

Washington, C. (2000). The challenge of adolescence pregnancy: The role of mother and father. In S. F. Battle (Ed.). The state of Black Milwaukee. Milwaukee, WI: Milwaukee Urban League, Inc., pp. 87-95.

Willis, E. (2000). Health disparities and children in Milwaukee. In S. F. Battle (Ed.). The state of Black Milwaukee. Milwaukee, WI: Milwaukee Urban League, Inc., pp. 57-80.

Wisconsin Department of Health and Family Services. (1998). Brighter futures: The Wisconsin plan to prevent adolescent pregnancy.

Wisconsin Department of Health and Social Services. (1990). Healthier people in Wisconsin: A public health agenda for the year 2000.

Child Support
and African American Teen Fathers

Judith L. Rozie-Battle, MSW, JD

SUMMARY. Our nation has turned its focus to personal responsibility and has subsequently formulated polices that have reformed welfare and strengthened child support enforcement. Teen fathers continue to present dilemmas for policy makers because of their status as minors, their lack of understanding of the policy implications for parenthood, their lack of skills, and their high unemployment status. African American teen fathers shoulder a larger burden in respect to the high unemployment rates and high drop out rates for African American males. Policies and programs must be developed that not only involve teen fathers with their children, but also provide them with the skills necessary to financially support themselves and their children. *[Article copies available for a fee from The Haworth Document Delivery Service: 1-800-HAWORTH. E-mail address: <getinfo@haworthpressinc.com> Website: <http://www.HaworthPress.com> © 2002 by The Haworth Press, Inc. All rights reserved.]*

KEYWORDS. African American, adolescent fathers, child support, paternity

African American teen parents account for a large number of the teen births in this nation. Young, unmarried fathers are rarely the focus in the

Judith L. Rozie-Battle is affiliated with the University of Wisconsin-Milwaukee, Helen Bader School of Social Welfare.

[Haworth co-indexing entry note]: "Child Support and African American Teen Fathers." Rozie-Battle, Judith L. Co-published simultaneously in *Journal of Health & Social Policy* (The Haworth Press, Inc.) Vol. 15, No. 2, 2002, pp. 45-58; and: *African-American Adolescents in the Urban Community: Social Services Policy and Practice Interventions* (ed: Judith L. Rozie-Battle) The Haworth Press, Inc., 2002, pp. 45-58. Single or multiple copies of this article are available for a fee from The Haworth Document Delivery Service [1-800-HAWORTH, 9:00 a.m. - 5:00 p.m. (EST). E-mail address: getinfo@haworthpressinc.com].

45

child support enforcement literature. A few articles discuss low-income fathers, (Turetsky, 2000; Edin, Lein, and Nelson, 1998) or absent fathers (Seltzer and Branchi, 1988), but they rarely discuss the consequences of child support enforcement efforts for adolescent fathers. The child support policies of this nation apply to these young men–as they do to all parents. Yet, there are special considerations that must be addressed for adolescent fathers.

PATERNITY

Paternity is defined as "the state or condition of a father, especially a biological one; fatherhood" (Garner, 1999). Several factors make paternity significant for both children and parents. Paternity adjudication goes beyond the traditional child support payments. It allows a child the opportunity to be eligible for other benefits, such as social security survivors or disability benefits, veteran's benefits, private insurance, inheritance rights, and property divisions following the death of a parent. (Everette, 1985). More importantly, if paternity is not established, a child will not be eligible for financial support through Temporary Assistance to Needy Families (TANF), food stamps, Medicaid, or other government benefits.

Paternity adjudication provides several rights to the father, which may include visitation, input on potential adoption, and involvement on major life and medical decisions for the child. Although we discuss fathers' rights and responsibilities as part of the outcome of paternity adjudication, these rights are often obscured by the economic responsibility.

Paternity can generally be established in two ways: through voluntary acknowledgment or through adjudication. The father can voluntarily sign the appropriate forms upon the birth of the child acknowledging that he is the father. If there is a disagreement between the mother and the putative father, either party can request a court hearing, usually referred to as a paternity action. A judge will make the determination whether a man is the father of a child based upon the evidence resulting from a paternity test. Paternity tests usually involve DNA identification or "tissue typing" to determine biological fatherhood.

Since it is common for the courts to determine custody and visitation orders following an adjudication of paternity, this would be an appropriate time for fathers interested in more involvement with their children to step forward and seek visitation orders. However, because the parties and the courts focus on child support payments and not the more personal issues affecting fathers, too often the process of establishing paternity creates anger and tensions between the parties and even the court. Fathers often see the support orders as additional support to the mother of the child and resent making the payments. If a father is unable to pay and the debt accumulates, the father may "end up in jail, and hostility and resentment will build toward mother and children as well as government authority (Johnson and Doolittle, 1998). It is also common practice that orders for child support and visitation are decided in separate courts before different judges or magistrates resulting in conflicting court decisions effecting individual families.

THE ROLE OF FATHERS

The role of the father has been subjugated in America. This limited role has been reinforced over the years in many circumstances, including the legal presumption referred to as the "tender years doctrine." This doctrine dates back to the late 1800s and early 1900s when fathers were still generally awarded custody of their children following divorce. In an effort to counter this one-sided practice, this doctrine was developed to take the needs of the children into consideration. The doctrine was a legal assumption that the well-being of children, particularly young children under the age of seven, would be better served by being placed with their mothers in any custody disputes. Although this doctrine has been abolished in almost every jurisdiction, the actions of individual judges and courts indicate it is still a common practice.

Traditionally, the father has not been viewed as a parent, instead he has been perceived as a spouse/partner for the mother of the child and as a financial resource. ". . . [E]xcept for his financial contribution, the father is a disposable parent" (McCant, 1987). In the case of young African American fathers, the financial contribution is usually lacking or so minuscule that he indeed is a disposable parent in the eyes of society (Rozie-Battle, 1990). The psychological message we send to young men is that the father is the perpetrator and the mother the victim (Battle, 1990).

This description has changed very little over the past twenty years. Despite changes in family compositions, between 1950 and 1994 the percentage of children living in mother-only families climbed from six percent to 24 percent (Blankenhorn, 1995). In recent years, there has been an increase in the number of fathers who choose to stay home and raise their children while the spouse/mother pursues her career. Despite this increase, the numbers of fathers involved with their children and sharing in the day to day rearing of their children are still the minority. The role of fathers continues to be defined generally in terms of financial contributions. This is particularly true for fathers of children receiving public support, as evidenced by the increased national child support enforcement efforts.

In his study of divorced fathers, Kruk found fathers disengage from their children soon after separation and that over time that disengagement increases. These fathers identified the loss of the father/child relationship as of the most salient factors in their transition. Those fathers who were close to their children felt more loss, while others found new ways to relate to their children and in fact adapted to the new role of part-time visiting dad (Kruk, 1994). Data from the National Commission on Children and other research supports the fact those fathers who do not live with their children loose contact with them over time (Seltzer, 1991). There is no reason to believe it would or should be any different for adolescent fathers. Fathers need to be nurtured in order to build healthy relationships with their families. When the father is connected with his child, emotional bonds are created and the home environment is affected (Ballard, 1998). For the sake of our children and the future, fathers must be seen as more than just financial providers.

There is a belief that a father who pays child support will desire to be involved with his children. The potential for increased involvement of fathers with their children may be an upside to the strict child support enforcement efforts. However, it would be fallacy to assume that every father who pays child support will automatically desire to spend more quality time with his children. Furthermore, in some circumstances there may be a need to be cautious about individual fathers having contact with their children, because it may not be in the best interest of the child. For example, in families where issues of violence or poor role modeling are present or are a major concern, safeguards must be put in place for the safety and well-being of the children. However, these situations should not be considered the norm and should not preclude encouraging fathers to be involved with their children. The bottom line is that in most situations, it is better for children to know and have contact with their fathers (Furstenberg, 1987; King, 1994).

The political environment in America today has swung toward less public assistance and more personal responsibility. This "mood" has allowed policy makers to introduce and implement legislation that increases efforts to collect child support payments from absent parents to support their children. Since fathers are overwhelmingly the absent parent, the psychological message sent to fathers is clear–pay or no contact. These subtle messages are often sent by child support enforcement officials, but more importantly, the mother of the children also relay these same messages. Although the legal issues of visitation and child support have theoretically been viewed as separate judicial determinations, in practice the two issues have not been so clearly severed. Fathers need assistance in understanding the importance of voluntarily contributing and being involved with their children. It will take new interventions and focused efforts on the part of support enforcement officials and social service organizations. These new methods are needed to assure fathers that the social service delivery system is supportive and receptive to their needs and not just as an extension of law enforcement.

CHILD SUPPORT

Child support becomes an issue for families when the parents divorce, never marry, or live apart. The issue of child support has become of critical importance to the government. It is seen as a way to reduce or recoup government dollars spent on the support of children whose parents do not live with or support them. Child support efforts have been challenging enough when parents live in the same state. However, when parents live in different states, the attempts to collect child support have been more complicated. Efforts by the federal government to improve the collection of support payments have lead to a number of federal requirements being imposed on the states in order to achieve this goal.

The National Conference of Commissioners on Uniform State Laws (NCCUSL) initiated the earliest efforts to establish uniform rules and policies concerning child support. This group drafted the Uniform Reciprocal Enforcement of Support Act (URESA) in 1950, which was subsequently adopted, in whole or in part, by most states. This voluntary act made it possible for a custodial parent in one state to obtain a court order in another state, where the non-custodial parent resided or owned property. This was an improvement because prior to this act, the custodial parent was required to travel to the noncustodial parent's state to initiate an action for child support.

Under URESA, there were two ways to obtain a valid court order. The first option was to register a court order from the custodial parent's state in the noncustodial parent's state, where it would be enforced. The second option was to file an interstate petition for a new order consistent with the guidelines of the noncustodial parent's state. In 1968, URESA was revised and became the Revised Uniform Reciprocal Enforcement of Support Act (RURESA), and by 1992 all states had adopted either URESA or RURESA. The problems encountered with both versions of this child support legislation were numerous. The problems included: the length of time for a petition to be heard; the possibility of two co-existing orders; the right of the non-custodial parent's state to modify an order of the custodial parent's state; and the inconsistency of enforcement efforts from state to state. These difficulties contributed to creating tensions and hostilities in the child support process.

During this period, Congress passed the Family Support Act of 1988. It required all states to develop a fully automated statewide child support system and mandated the states' to review and modify, if necessary, all child support orders for families receiving public assistance at least every 36 months (P.L. 100-485, 1988).

The most recent policy enacted by the federal government to enforce child support payments is the Uniform Interstate Family Support Act of 1992 (UIFSA) and its 1996 amendments. UIFSA provided for only one controlling support order; included a broad long-arm provision; allowed a wage withholding order to be sent directly to an out-of-state-employer, and contained detailed provisions governing a two-state process (Department of Health and Human Services, 2000).

In 1996, Congress passed the Personal Responsibility and Work Opportunity Reconciliation Act (PRWORA), which made sweeping changes to the federally funded welfare programs in this nation. Although not specifically child support legislation, it did require states to adopt UIFSA and contained mandates to qualify for federal funding. In order to continue receiving federal funds for child support enforcement and public assistance programs, states were required to designate one state agency to implement and monitor child support statewide. States were also required to put in place procedures related to child support systems and the establishment of paternity by specified deadlines. The PRWORA included provisions to strengthen withholding orders and the establishment of a "new hire" reporting system, whereby employers were required to report all new hires to the designated state support enforcement agency (P.L. 104-193, 1996).

PRWORA also included several provisions specifically aimed at teen parents, although most were directed at mothers. Under PRWORA, states must develop alternative sites for the establishment of voluntary paternity, provide information explaining the rights and responsibilities of minor parents, and inform the young parents of any state laws that protect them as minor parents. States treat these practices differently so there is no consistency in the application of the law. For example, in California a minor father can sign the documents establishing paternity, but this information cannot be used for child support collection until the young man is legally an adult at age 18 (Levin-Epstein, 1996).

The NCCUSL has recently revised and approved the Uniform Parentage Act of 2000 (UPA), which provides guidance to the states on determining parenthood. The revised UPA consolidates for the states' eligibility provisions required by the federal government in order to receive federal dollars (CLASP, 2000). It is expected that most states will adopt all of portions of the revised act.

In addition, Congress has introduced the Child Support Distribution Act of 2000, which has passed the House of Representatives and is expected to pass in the Senate. This act includes provisions for the distribution of grants for community services that improve the ability of fathers to support their children. The Department of Heath and Human Services–Fatherhood Initiative, is an example of a policy that is developing programs and other supportive efforts for fathers, and expanding the services to the local level.

Each of the previously mentioned federal laws required all states to establish guidelines and procedures for child support awards that applied to all noncustodial parents. There was no exception in any of the legislation for young, poor, or disabled fathers. The government's desire to recoup money for children whose custodial parent received public assistance is both apparent and understandable. Paternity establishment services are mandated for families receiving public assistance, although the services are available for any family regardless of income, through the designated child support agency. Many of the fathers of children receiving public assistance have limited income themselves. It is unclear what the expectations are, in terms of realized income, on the part of policy makers. "Expecting these men to reimburse past welfare payments made by federal and state governments to their children, over and above their child support obligations established by the state is a recipe for failure" (Johnson and Doolittle, 1998).

AFRICAN AMERICAN ADOLESCENT FATHERS

An adolescent male who becomes a father is expected to embody the father role while he is still negotiating the developmental tasks of adolescents. Depending upon his own cognitive and psychosocial development, he may or may not be able to provide emotional support for a young mother and contribute to the nurturance of their offspring.

In addition, several prejudicial social factors, including the economic and social welfare systems, exclude adolescent fathers from continuing the relationship with their partners and actively participating in their children's upbringing. Often the adolescent father is unmarried and physically separated at the time of the child's birth and early childhood, thereby reducing the number of opportunities available for interaction with the infant. These young men often encounter rejection and anger from the mother of the child resulting in limited contact with the child. They may also fear they are unable to provide financial support and may face rejection from other family members (Knitzer and Bernard, 1997). A teen father's absence leads to a common misconception of not caring among health care providers who often perceive adolescent fathers as irresponsible deserters of their children. The divorce rate for adolescent parents is five times higher than for adults (Panzarine and Elster, 1982). The unrealistic expectations of adolescent mothers about the father's marriage plans, coupled with the reality that most adolescent fathers are not interested in marriage, may further contribute to the negative view of the adolescent father so prevalent in the literature (Battle, 1999). In fact, many young fathers believe they are not prepared for fatherhood and have difficulty assuming the responsibilities at this stage of their development (Kahn and Bolton, 1986).

There is a disconnection between what young fathers think they know and what they actually know. Adolescent fathers lack a clear understanding of the child support enforcement laws and the applicability of these laws to them.

Young men need to realize that fatherhood during adolescence makes them subject to support obligations until the child is at least eighteen years of age. Efforts for child support enforcement have been strengthened over the past ten years and many young men believe that because in prior years they were not required to provide support, they will not be required to do so in the future. They also believe that if they are unemployed they will not be held accountable for child support payments. Finally, they do not understand that if they do not pay child support from the time the child is born, they can be held responsible for past payments. The payment of these arrearages can occur when they obtain a job or acquire a better paying job in the future. African American young men must be made aware of the laws that are designed to ensure that children are supported by both parents.

Much of the child support enforcement effort focuses on withholding income from fathers to support their children. For many young fathers, this is difficult because of age or skill levels. Based on statistics from 1999, the U.S. Labor Department, unemployment rates for young White men between the ages of 16 and 21 were 13%, while African American men of the same age range experienced an unemployment rate of 31%. Consequently, many young African American fathers are able to pay little toward child support, if anything at all (U. S. Department of Labor, 1999). As Jeff Johnson of the National Center for Strategic Non-Profit Planning and Community Leadership in Washington, D.C., has said, "these dads are dead broke, not dead beat."

Young fathers have the option of having a judgment reserved or a minimal order put in place, while they are still in school, unemployed, or able to work only part-time. Unfortunately, many young men are not aware of this option and consequently do not take advantage of it. This option does not free the young father from supporting his children, but does allow him to make a reasonable effort, with the understanding that as his income increases, the order will be adjusted accordingly.

Some states have not enforced delinquent child support payments on minor fathers, while others, such as Texas, have prosecuted minor fathers for failure to pay child support (Levin-Epstein, 1996). Other states have taken a stronger position and enacted "grandparent liability" statutes to ensure financial support for children born to teen fathers. Wisconsin, for example has a statute that provides that if a young man is under the age of eighteen and in school, the court may order his parents to help with the support of the grandchild (Wis. Stat.§, 49.90, 1999-00). This statute is an example of the policies that many young men and their parents are commonly unaware of or do not fully understand the ramifications. It is important to note the application of this law is uneven, resulting in inconsistent enforcement. Finally, some states have developed community services obligations for minor fathers in lieu of child support (Levin-Epstein, 1996).

Information regarding paternity and child support enforcement efforts are critical for young men to assist them in making decisions regarding sexual activity and potential fatherhood. The families of these young men, the Black churches, schools, and community social service organizations that work with young parents must include fathers and provide them with the knowledge to help them make informed and responsible decisions (Rozie-Battle, 1990). Prevention programs that reach young men prior to them becoming fathers are most critical. Educational and support programs that begin early and are honest, factual, and straightforward are most likely to benefit young men.

IMPLICATIONS FOR PRACTITIONERS
AND POLICY MAKERS

Although there has been an increase in the number of programs that serve adolescent fathers, the numbers remain relatively small. Some programs claim to work with "young parents," but when looking at their goals, objectives, and services, they are clearly focused on the young mother and/or the child. The focus of many adolescent parenting programs are twofold: primary prevention and support services (Hofferth, 1991). Unfortunately, most programs continue to focus their efforts on the young mother. Prevention programs can be further divided into primary and secondary prevention services. Primary prevention services are those programs designed to prevent first pregnancies, and secondary prevention services focus on the prevention of subsequent pregnancies (Franklin and Corcoran, 2000).

Both types of prevention programs are critical for young African American fathers. The prevention of initial pregnancies and the issue of subsequent pregnancies with young men as well as young women must be addressed.

Many fathers provide for their children through methods other than formal cash support payments. The "pamper defense" is one that refers to the type of support many young fathers feel is acceptable and attainable for them. When asked whether they support their children, many young fathers say, they purchase "pampers" and clothes. Yet, our system has not developed a means of taking these types of contributions into account. Waller and Plotnick (2000), refer to these donations and noncash contributions as in-kind donations. The Internal Revenue Service provides for and allows nonprofit organizations to count and credit organizations and individuals for in-kind contributions, but we have yet to figure out how to do this for young fathers, and in many cases poor fathers. This is not to say that these noncash contributions are sufficient or the only contributions needed to raise a child, but they may be the only contributions these young men can realistically make at this point in their lives. This is particularly true for young African American teen fathers between the ages of 16 and 25 who have such high unemployment rates.

Policy makers and program directors need to work toward policies that look at the true potential of fathers. This is particularly true in the poorer and culturally diverse communities in America. Examples include, strengthening existing support enforcement programs to assist young fathers with job training programs and completion of high school or a GED. Services should be readily available and not restricted solely to those with TANF eligibility. Although some states are beginning to untangle the TANF eligibility and job training eligibility, it is neither consistent nor sufficient in practice.

Utilization of community and technical colleges are an inexpensive and focused method of obtaining concrete skills and training for young fathers, and many are conveniently located in the urban areas.

The delivery of services needs to be revamped to focus on supportive services, including outreach and a friendly environment, as opposed to approaching the services from a victim/perpetrator mentality.

Further development and an increase in the intensity of community education programs, similar to those used in HIV and substance abuse efforts in the minority community should be considered. By determining what has worked in those venues could be a model for pregnancy prevention programs for young African American men.

Finally, we must determine which existing programs are most effective and replicate them as much as possible. For example, outcomes based research provides some guidance for the type of programs that are most effective. The general findings indicate that community based clinics are more effective than school-based clinics (Franklin and Corcoran, 2000).

As an international leader among nations, the United States needs to better educate and inform young people, both male and female, as well as their parents/guardians of the rights and responsibilities of parenthood. They must be informed about the law and the effect the law may have on them. Policies must be written in plain language so that the average person affected by them can understand what is being said and how it applies to them. Parents and/or guardians must be aware of the consequences for them personally, as the parents of adolescents who may become parents early.

Youth development programming must incorporate the consequences of having children early. To focus solely on the issue of abstinence limits the development of young people and deprives them of the information they need regarding the rights, responsibilities, and consequences for early parenthood. The opportunity to make choices through informed consent is critical for the development of young African American men and for a successful prevention effort.

Policy makers must look at methods of encouraging payments early and regularly, even if the payments are small. Setting payments at realistic levels that fathers can attain will assist fathers in making and maintaining their payment schedules (Turetsky, 2000).

Policy makers further need to understand the needs of the community and the people who are affected by the decisions they make. Advisory groups of young people need to have input on the policies. This process will help develop young people into productive adults and community members who feel they have a stake in the prevention efforts. Use of peer leaders and peer counselors can also be a productive use of young people in the effort to stem early parenthood.

CONCLUSION

Adolescent African American fathers must be recognized and respected, not just for the financial support they may be able to provide, but for the psychological and emotional support they can provide for their children and the stability of the community. A review of current policies to determine how consistent these policies conform with the capabilities and realities of young fathers is important, particularly in light of the earning power of young African American men between the ages 16-21. The impact current policies have on young African American fathers in terms of fostering relationships with their children must be reviewed.

Paternity adjudication and child support procedures and policies need to be reviewed and made more flexible and consumer friendly. Policies and programs should encourage noncustodial fathers, particularly young fathers, to seek out services to assist them with providing financial support for their children. These programs should also provide supportive and culturally-sensitive services to fathers who desire more involvement with their children.

Finally, policy makers and the courts must look beyond the legal issues of establishing paternity and financial support for children. Although this is certainly a critical step, the strengthening and funding of community services that can assist young African American fathers in attaining the skills necessary for employment are just as critical. The ability to provide for a child financially will help young men be more confident and personally involved in the lives of their children.

REFERENCES

Ballard, J. (1998). *Institute for responsible fatherhood and family revitalization.* Cleveland, OH.

Barrett, R.L. and Robinson, B.E. (1982). Teenage fathers: Neglected too long. *Social Work,* 11, 484-488.

Battle, S. (1987). Key informant, *Adolescent pregnancy: Problems and prospects.* Massachusetts Somerville Producers Group, Cable Access Television.

Battle, S. (Ed.) (1999). *The state of Black Milwaukee,* Milwaukee, WI: Milwaukee Urban League, Inc.

Blankenhorn, D. (1995). *Fatherless America: Confronting our most urgent social problems.* New York: Bais Books.

Coleman, M., Ganong, L., Killian, T. and McDaniel, A. (1999). Child support obligations, attitudes and rationale. *Journal of Family Issues,* 20(1), 46-68.

Edin, K., Lein, L., and Nelson, T. (1998). Low-income non-residential fathers: Off balance in a competitive economy: An initial analysis. Washington, D.C.: Department of Health and Human Services Fatherhood Initiative.

Everett, J.E. (1985). An examination of child support enforcement issues, in Harriet McAdoo and T.M. Jim Parnham (Eds.), *Services to young families,* Washington D.C.: American Public Welfare Association.

Family Support Act of 1988. *Public Law No. 100-485,* 102 Stat. 2843.

Franklin, C. and Corcoran, J. (2000). Preventing adolescent pregnancy: A review of programs and practices. *Social Work,* Vol. 45(1), 40-52.

Furstenberg, F. (1999). Sexual partners and their children. *Journal of Marriage and Family,* 2, 74-84.

Furstenberg, Jr. F., Morgan, S.P., and Allison, P.D. (1987). Paternal participation and children's well-being. *American Sociological Review,* 52, 695-701.

Garner, B.A. (Ed.) (1999). *Black's law dictionary,* 7th edition, St. Paul, MN: West Publishing Company.

Henricks, L.E. (1988). Outreach with teenage fathers: A preliminary report on three ethnic groups. *Adolescence,* 23, 711-723.

Hofferth, S.H. (1991). Programs for high-risk adolescents. *Evaluation and Program Planning.* 14, 3-16.

Johnson E.S. and Doolittle, F. (1998). Low income parents and parent's fair share program: An early qualitative look at one public policy initiative's attempt to improve the ability and desire of low income noncustodial parents to pay child support. In I. Garfinkle, S. McLanahan, D. Meyer, and J. Seltzer, *Fathers under fire: the revolution in child support enforcement.* Russell Sage Foundation, Chapter 9.

Kahn, J.S., and Bolton, F.G., Jr. (1986). Clinical issues in adolescent fatherhood. In A.B. Elster and M.E. Lamb, *Adolescent fatherhood,* Hillsdale, NJ: Erlbaum.

King, V. (1994). Nonresidential father involvement and child well-being: Can dads make a difference? *Journal of Family Issues* 15, 78-96.

Knitzer, J. and Bernard, S. (1997). Map and track: State initiatives to encourage responsible fatherhood. New York: National Center on Children in Poverty.

Kruk, E. (1994). The disengaged noncustodial father: Implications for social work practice with the divorced family. *Social Work,* 139(1), 15-24.

Levin-Epstein, J. (1996). Teen parent provisions in the Personal Responsibility and Work Opportunity Act of 1996. Washington, D.C.: The Center for Law and Social Policy.

McCant, J. (1987). The cultural contradictions of fathers as nonparents. *Family Law Quarterly*, 21(3), 127-143.

Miller, D. (1997). Adolescent fathers: What we know and what we need to know. *Child and Adolescence Social Work Journal*, 14, 66-69.

Panzarine, S. and Elster, A.B. (1982). Prospective adolescent father: Stresses during pregnancy and implication for nursing interventions. *Journal of Psychosocial Nursing and Mental Health Services*, 200(7), 21-24.

Personal Responsibility and Work Opportunity Reconciliation Act of 1996. *Public Law 104-193*, 110 Stat.2105.

Robinson, B.E. (1988). Teenage pregnancy from the father's perspective. *American Journal of Orthopsychiatry*, 58, 46-51.

Rozie-Battle, J. (1990). Adolescent fathers: The question of paternity. In D. Jones and S. Battle (Eds.). *Teenage pregnancy-developing strategies for change in the twenty-first century*. New Brunswick, NJ: Transaction Publishers.

Rozie-Battle, J. (1995). Key informant. Focus groups with adolescent fathers, Asylum Hill Organizing Project, Summer Youth League, Hartford, CT.

Seltzer, J.A. (1991). Relationships between fathers and children who live apart: The father's role after separation. *Journal of Marriage and The Family*, 53:79-101.

Seltzer, J.A., and Branchi S.M. (1988). Children in contact with absent parents. *Journal of Marriage and The Family*, 50:663-677.

Sorenson, E. and Zibma, C. (2000). Child support offers some protection against poverty. *New Federalism*, Series B, B-10, Washington, D.C.: The Urban Institute.

Turetsky, V. (2000). Realistic child support policies for low-income fathers. Kellogg Devolution Initiative Paper, Washington, D.C.: Center for Law and Social Policy.

U.S. Labor Department. Retrieved March 20, 1999 from the World Wide Web (http://www.146.142.4.24./cgi_bin/surveymost).

U. S. Department of Health and Human Services. Retrieved February 7, 2000 from the World Wide Web (www.acf.dhhs.gov/programs/cse/pol/dc119814.htm).

Waller, M. and Plotnick, R. (2000). A failed relationship? Low-income families and the child support enforcement system. *Focus*, 21(1).Wis. Stat. §, 49.90, 1999-00.

African American Girls
and the Challenges Ahead

Judith L. Rozie-Battle, MSW, JD

SUMMARY. The research on the psychosocial development of African American girls is limited. Information that is available focuses on teen pregnancy and health issues such as nutrition and physical activity. African American girls are facing challenges, including poverty, crime, poor self-esteem, and peer pressure. Despite some of the negative characteristics attributed to African American girls, many are achieving some success. Policy makers and service providers need to recognize the resiliency and unique needs of African American girls and develop services that ensure their needs are being fully met. *[Article copies available for a fee from The Haworth Document Delivery Service: 1-800-HAWORTH. E-mail address: <getinfo@haworthpressinc.com> Website: <http://www.HaworthPress.com> © 2002 by The Haworth Press, Inc. All rights reserved.]*

KEYWORDS. African American girls, resiliency, religious involvement, service delivery

INTRODUCTION

Literature on youth, particularly African American youth, focuses on negative behaviors and attitudes. Publications specifically examining the needs of adolescent African American girls are limited, with the exceptions

Judith L. Rozie-Battle is affiliated with the University of Wisconsin-Milwaukee, Helen Bader School of Social Welfare.

[Haworth co-indexing entry note]: "African American Girls and the Challenges Ahead." Rozie-Battle, Judith L. Co-published simultaneously in *Journal of Health & Social Policy* (The Haworth Press, Inc.) Vol. 15, No. 2, 2002, pp. 59-67; and: *African-American Adolescents in the Urban Community: Social Services Policy and Practice Interventions* (ed: Judith L. Rozie-Battle) The Haworth Press, Inc., 2002, pp. 59-67. Single or multiple copies of this article are available for a fee from The Haworth Document Delivery Service [1-800-HAWORTH, 9:00 a.m. - 5:00 p.m. (EST). E-mail address: getinfo@haworthpressinc.com].

of the high volumes of literature concerning teen sexuality and preg-nancy (Dixon, Schoonmaker, and Philliber, 2000; East, 1998; Corcoran and Kunz, 1997); and health and wellness concerns, such as nutrition and physical activity, usually in comparison to their White counterparts (Grant, Lyons, Landis, Cho, Scudiero, Reynolds, Murphy, and Bryant, 1999; Halpern, Udry, Campbell, and Suchindran, 1999).

Many urban African American girls today face challenges their mothers and grandmothers were not confronted with. These girls are ex-pected to endure a more sexually permissive society and a world that is overtly more violent toward women. The daily harassment of female students at school, in conjunction with the high incidence of sexual abuse against females, are indications that there are few safe places for young women today (Davis, 1999). In a national report by the Carnegie Council on Adolescent Development (1995), the findings indicated that one fourth of adolescents between the ages of ten and sixteen reported they were the victim of a sexual assault in the previous year.

Young women today also face high levels of teen pregnancy, ele-vated HIV/AIDS rates, and other sexually transmitted diseases (STDs). The escalation of violence in their homes, schools, and communities is well documented. There is more competition than ever before in the ed-ucational system and the workplace as a result of changes in the politi-cal environment.

Adolescents are torn between the desire to belong and be accepted by their peers and the pressure from peers to participate in negative behav-iors, such as the use alcohol and drugs. For many African American youth, there is also pressure from family to follow the cultural tradition of involvement in the church or some form of organized religion. While many African American youth remain involved and spiritually con-nected, too many are rejecting this cultural tradition as irrelevant and out-of-date.

Efforts by African American students to achieve recognition as seri-ous students are often belittled by others and create feelings of self-con-sciousness on the part of some. Those who are achieving feel isolated and ignored unless they are able to connect with positive programs in the community that respect their abilities and utilize their skills.

These are just a few of the key dilemmas youth face today. For Afri-can American girls the dilemmas can be more compelling because the Black female experience defies a singular definition. "For instance, counterpoised to the image of the teenage single mother is the concept of the strong, enduring Black women as an historical type" (Davis,

1999). This statement is indicative of the dual perspective that young girls today experience.

There is a great deal of pressure exerted on young women to achieve and to support the African American family and the community. Yet, for too many young women, early parenthood or poor academics do not allow them to reach this goal. Once they become parents at an early age they are besieged with the risk of dropping out of school and a future of poverty.

This paper will provide a glimpse of four areas of challenge for urban African American girls today: self-esteem, resiliency, the church, and juvenile crime. It will also examine how service providers and policy makers can develop more successful interventions and outcomes with the African American girls of the 21st century.

THE STATUS OF AFRICAN AMERICAN GIRLS

The majority of the literature on African American youth focuses on males and the crisis of the male, however young women are "also experiencing a crisis, although it is less likely to express itself in involvement in the criminal justice system, and more likely to express itself in a variety of other destructive, opportunity-constraining behaviors, such as increased likelihood of adolescent pregnancy (Brown, 2000). African American adolescent females utilize more self directed destructions. It does not mean that females will not become involved in some of the same activities as males, but as a group, females are less likely to be involved in some of the more serious criminal activities.

Self-Esteem

Issues of self-esteem for African American girls are quite complex and range from the impact of family functioning to personal acceptance of self.

Family functioning plays a significant role in the development of positive self-esteem for African American girls. From a study by Mandara and Murray (2000), it was reported that positive family functioning had more effect on the self esteem of teen African American girls than did the marital status of the family. In other words, regardless of whether an African American girl is from a single parent or a two-parent family home, a positive relationship with her parent(s) is more critical to her positive self-development. Despite the high number of single parent families within the African American community, that fact alone is not the most important issue in the development of a girl's self-esteem.

Further, in the area of personal acceptance there have been several studies that deal with issues of "beauty" or appearance. Overall, the "acceptable" beauty standard of the mainstream has been one that depicted the characteristics of Caucasian females, as opposed to women of color. In a study of the effects of media on White and minority girls, researchers found that minority girls do not identify with "White" media images, nor believe that significant others are effected by them (Milkie, 1999). Consequently, the study indicated that Black girls were refuting images that present the White beauty standard as the norm. In another study on the impact of teen magazines on teen girls, it was found that while Black girls read the mainstream magazines, they do so for "generic content on topics like social issues and entertainment" and in general they expressed little interest in the magazines "beauty images because they conflicted with African American standards of attractiveness" (Duke, 2000).

These studies appear to be consistent with a 1995 study by the University of Arizona which found that 70% of African American teens are satisfied with their bodies (Davis, 1999). These studies indicate a denial of the acceptance of White beauty as the standard by African American girls. However, for some African American girls, there is a pressure to meet the White beauty myth. The pressure can be more intense for some girls due to competition based on hair texture, skin complexion, and intellectual capacity. Among urban African American girls, there are vast differences based on class and levels of assimilation attributed to young women. Each of these factors also plays into the identification with mainstream beauty.

Resiliency

The research on resiliency focuses on mechanisms or factors that "enhance resiliency of disadvantaged groups over various stages of their life development" (Hill, 1998). Hill developed a resiliency framework that describes protective mechanisms at three ecological levels–individual, family, and community. For teen girls, all three levels are critical to their overall development.

The resiliency of young girls despite the many pressures they experience is evident in two recent projects that focused on African American girls and youth.

In a study of 30 Black girls, aged 14-19, residing in the inner city, the findings indicated that overall the girls were hopeful, despite their fear of violence. There was some indication in the findings that violence negatively affected their hopefulness, but the impact was not clear. These girls expressed a shared value of mainstream society in terms of future aspirations and assessments of their communities (Brown and Gourdine, 1998).

In a book entitled *The State of Black Milwaukee Through the Eyes of Children,* several middle and high school students wrote essays about violence in their community, schools, and their future plans. Despite some of the bleak attributes of the metropolitan community in which they resided, several common themes emerged for the students, the vast majority of whom were female. They aspired to have academic success, which included definite plans for higher education, they expressed concern about the levels of drug and alcohol use in their communities, and concern about the violence in their schools and communities. Several of the young women also spoke strongly about inter- and intra-racial harmony. Finally, a majority of the students indicated a strong sense of faith and spirituality.

In terms of career aspirations, the girls indicated they had specific goals that ranged from entrepreneurs to teachers. They also discussed clear educational steps to help them achieve their future goals. The vast majority of the girls were from the inner city of Milwaukee and it is a city with many of the typical urban characteristics. Yet, these young people were able to identify key people they felt could assist them in their plans, including, supportive parents, extended family members, teachers, and a strong spiritual foundation (Rozie-Battle and Battle, 1999).

Although these findings reflect a small number of young women, they are at least an initial look at how young women are responding to the struggles they endure daily.

The Role of the Church

The Black church has had a long tradition in the African American community. Despite concerns by some that African American youth are straying from those roots, research indicates that African American youth attend formal services more frequently than European Americans, and this finding is consistent with earlier research which reflects a stronger religious orientation for African Americans (Markstrom, 1999).

There have been several studies since 1986 that have examined the impact of church/religious involvement on the level of crime among youth (Freeman, 1986; Johnson, Larson, Li, and Jang, 2000). These studies each indicate that religious involvement has a negative effect on criminal activities of African American male teens. For girls, religious involvement has been shown to have a limited impact as a protective factor on crime (Grant, O'Koon, Davis et al., 2000). Young women who are involved in some form of organized religion are less likely than their peers to become involved in the juvenile justice system.

Based on the findings of these studies, over the past fifteen years, it is clear that the Black church can and must play an important role in the development of African American youth.

Crime and Gangs

Several recent reports indicate that the crime rate for Black adolescent girls has increased by 50% between 1968 and 1994 (Molidor, 1996) and despite a recent decrease in the overall crime rate by teens, there has been an increase in the rate of crime among girls (Snyder and Sickmund, 1999). Of more concern is the increase of serious crime among girls (Taylor, 1993), including homicide and drug trafficking.

Peer pressure is believed to have the largest influence on gang involvement for females. Girls turn to gangs for protection not only from other gangs, but also from community violence and abusive families. Involvement in the gangs also provided girls with access to money that is not available through traditional social institutions. It is also a way of gaining respect (Walker-Barnes and Mason, 2001). Furthermore, gang involvement may be the result of the vulnerable status of adolescent females today. As victims of sexual harassment and sexual abuse, they may turn to the gang as a substitute family and protector.

IMPLICATIONS

The poverty rates in this country continue to show Black women in worse shape than their White counterparts. The overall poverty rates for Black women were approximately 29%, while the rates for Black females under the age of 18 were at 37% (McKinnon and Humes, 1999).

Currently, of the 8.4 million Black families in this country, less than one-half (47%) of all Black families were married-coupled families; 45% were maintained by women with no spouse; and 8% were Black men with no spouse (McKinnon and Humes, 1999). In the area of educational attainment, similar proportions of Black men and women 25 years of age and older were at least high school graduates; however, Black women were more likely to have completed at least a bachelor's degree (16% versus 14%).

Finally in the area of labor force unemployment, Black men and women continue to outpace their White counterparts. During the 1970s and 1980s, African American women experienced higher rates of employment and educational opportunities due to the emphasis on affirmative action and equal opportunity efforts. Because African American women could fill two "quotas"–female and Black, many employers and institutions of higher education sought African American women for employment and admissions. The negative turn of events in policy–the desire to dismantle affirmative action, has caused backlash for all African Americans, regardless of gender.

The data continues to point out the need for young African American women to continue to work toward maximum educational and job skills preparation.

Young African American women, expect to get their education, get married, have children, and live out the American dream, not unlike their White counterparts. When we consider the high levels of African American males who are incarcerated, addicted, or dead, the available pool of life partners shrinks considerably. Some young women may choose never to marry or may marry outside their race, but for those who do, the road can be challenging.

Social service providers must begin to look to one of the most enduring institutions in the African American community, the Black church, as a partner in their efforts to reach out to youth, particularly girls. Women have always had a strong role in the church and young women must be encouraged to participate as well. Involvement in the church and the community in general will assist in the development of positive self-esteem and productive skills.

Interventions with African American girls should be community- and faith-based. Outreach and service strategies should be geared toward all ages, but particularly middle and high school girls.

Efforts need to be made to address issues of intra-racial conflict over physical appearance, such as skin complexion and hair texture. Educational programs that instill a sense of pride in the African American culture and its history would assist young women to learn to support and respect one another and to end the tensions that exist between too many young women today.

Finally, providers must be cognizant of the pressures young women are under and create environments that are not hostile or threatening, but supportive and safe.

CONCLUSION

African American girls today have multiple challenges ahead of them. This nation must begin to understand the pressures that young women are experiencing and begin to develop and explore better options for meeting their needs. African American women have historically been strong contributors to the development of the African American community and this younger generation must be prepared to carry on that tradition.

REFERENCES

Brown, A.W. and Gourdine, R.M. (1998). Teenage Black girls and violence: Coming of age in an urban environment. *Journal of Human Behavior in the Social Environment*, Vol. 1, Nos. 2/3.

Brown, E. (2000). Black like me? "Gangsta" culture, Clarence Thomas, and Afrocentric academies. *New York University Law Review*, 75(20):308-353.

Carnegie Council on Adolescent Development. (1995). *Great transitions: Preparing adolescents for a new century.* Concluding Report. New York, NY: Carnegie Corporation.

Corcoran M. E. and Kunz, J. P. (1997). Do unmarried births among African American teens lead to adult poverty? *Social Service Review*, 71(2), 274-287.

Davis, N. J. (1999). *Youth crisis: Growing up in the high-risk society.* Westport, CT: Praeger.

Dixon, A. C., Schoonmaker, C. T. and Philliber, W.W. (2000). A journey toward womanhood: Effects of an Afrocentric approach to pregnancy prevention among African American adolescent females. *Adolescence*, 35(139), 425-429.

Duke, L. (2000). Black in a blond world: Race and girls interpretations of the feminine ,ideal in teen magazines. *Journal of Mass Communication Quarterly*, 77(2), 367-392.

East, P. L. (1998). Racial and ethnic differences in girls' sexual, marital, and birth expectations. *Journal of Marriage and Family* 60(1), 150-162.

Freeman, R. B. (1986). Who escapes? The relation of churchgoing and other background factors to the socioeconomic performance of Black males youth from inner-city tracts, In R. B. Freeman and H. J. Helzer (Eds). *The Black youth employment crisis.* Chicago, IL: University of Chicago Press.

Grant, K. Lyons, A., Landis, D., Cho, M. H., Scudiero, M., Reynolds, L., Murphy, J., and Bryant, H. (1999). Gender body image, and depressive symptoms among low-income African American adolescents. *Journal of Social Issues*, 55(2), 299-315.

Grant, K. E., O'Koon, J. H., Davis, T. H., Roache, N. A., Poindexter, L. M., Armstrong, M. L., Minden, J. A., and McIntosh, J. M. (2000). Protective factors affecting low-income urban African American youth exposed to stress. *Journal of Early Adolescence*, 20(4), 388-417.

Halpern, C. T., Udry, J. R., Campbell, B., and Suchindran, C. (1999). Effects of body fat on weight concerns, dating, and sexual activity: A longitudinal analysis of black and white adolescent girls. *Developmental Psychology*, 35(3), 721-736.

Hill, R. B. (1998). Enhancing the resilience of African American families. *Journal of Human Behavior in the Social Environment*, Vol. 1, Nos. 2/3.

Johnson, B. R., Larson, D. B., Li, D. D., and Jang, S. J. (2000). Escaping from the crime of inner cities: Church attendance and religious salience among disadvantaged youth. *Justice Quarterly*, 17:377-392.

Mandara, J. and Murray, C. B. (2000). Effect of parental marital status, income, and family functioning on African American adolescent self-esteem. *Journal of Family Psychology*, 14(3), 475-490.

Markstrom, C. (1999). Religious involvement and adolescent psychosocial development. *Journal of Adolescence*, 22:205-221.

McKinnon, J. and Humes, K. (1999). *The Black Population in the United States, 1999.* U. S. Census Bureau Current Populations Reports, Series P20-530. Washington, D.C.: U. S. Government Printing Office.

Milkie, M. A. (1999). Social comparisons, reflected appraisals, and mass media: The impact of pervasive beauty images on black ad white girls' self concepts. *Social Psychology Quarterly*, 62(2), 190-210.

Molidor, C. E. (1996). Female gang members: A profile of aggression and victimization, *Social Work*, 41(3), 251-257.

Rozie-Battle, J. and Battle, S. (Eds.) (1999). *The state of Black Milwaukee through the eyes of children.* Milwaukee, WI: Milwaukee Urban League, Inc.

Snyder, H. N. and Sickmund, M. (1999). *Juvenile offenders and victims:1999 national report.* Washington, D.C.: Office of Juvenile Justice and Delinquency Prevention, U.S. Department of Justice.

Taylor, C. S. (1993). Female: A historical perspective. In C. S. Taylor (Ed.), *Girls, gangs, women, and drugs.* East Lansing: Michigan State University Press, 13-47.

Walker-Barnes, C. J. and Mason, C. A. (2001). Perceptions of risk factors for female gang involvement among African American and Hispanic women. *Youth and Society*, 32(3), 303-336.

African American Teens
and the Neo-Juvenile Justice System

Judith L. Rozie-Battle, MSW, JD

SUMMARY. African American youth continue to be overrepresented in the juvenile justice system. As a result of the current political environment and the perceived increase in crime among young people, the nation has moved away from rehabilitation and toward harsher treatment of delinquents. The African American community must encourage policy makers and community leaders to continue to address the disproportionate representation of African American youth in the system. Current policing and prosecutorial policies must also be examined and challenged to end the perception of an unjust system. *[Article copies available for a fee from The Haworth Document Delivery Service: 1-800-HAWORTH. E-mail address: <getinfo@haworthpressinc.com> Website: <http://www.HaworthPress.com> © 2002 by The Haworth Press, Inc. All rights reserved.]*

KEYWORDS. Juvenile justice, waivers, African American, disproportionate representation

INTRODUCTION

Communities have raised concerns about the perceived increase in serious juvenile crime over the past five years. Many have believed that with an increase in the youthful population, there would be a related in-

Judith L. Rozie-Battle is affiliated with the University of Wisconsin-Milwaukee, Helen Bader School of Social Welfare.

[Haworth co-indexing entry note]: "African American Teens and the Neo-Juvenile Justice System." Rozie-Battle, Judith L. Co-published simultaneously in *Journal of Health & Social Policy* (The Haworth Press, Inc.) Vol. 15, No. 2, 2002, pp. 69-79; and: *African-American Adolescents in the Urban Community: Social Services Policy and Practice Interventions* (ed: Judith L. Rozie-Battle) The Haworth Press, Inc., 2002, pp. 69-79. Single or multiple copies of this article are available for a fee from The Haworth Document Delivery Service [1-800-HAWORTH, 9:00 a.m. - 5:00 p.m. (EST). E-mail address: getinfo@haworthpressinc.com].

crease in serious juvenile crime. According to the Children's Defense Fund, there has been a 23% overall decrease in the juvenile violent criminal arrest rate over a 5 year period from 1995-1999. This decrease in violent juvenile crime has occurred despite continuous growth in the youth population (Children's Defense Fund, 2000).

However, in the same five year period, 47 states plus the District of Columbia have enacted more punitive laws for their respective juvenile justice systems. Of the 47 states, 45 have enacted laws to make it easier to transfer a juvenile offender from the juvenile justice system to the adult criminal justice system, and all 47 have modified or removed laws that protect the confidentiality of juvenile court record and proceedings (Synder and Sickmund, 1999). These modifications have been based on a small percentage of high profile cases and the resulting backlash from communities.

In 1996, the juvenile courts in the United States handled an estimated 1.8 million cases in which the juvenile was charged with a delinquency (Synder and Sickmund, 1999). This distinction is important, because most juvenile justice systems also handle abuse and neglect cases as well as status offense cases, which are not included in these delinquency figures. From all indications, the juvenile court is an overburdened system.

The number of identified juvenile offenders between the ages of 14-17 increased between 1984 and 1993, but began to decline between 1994 and 1997 for all age groups. While the number of homicides committed by young men in the past decade fluctuated from a high in 1994 to about 1,600 in 1997, the number of homicides for females remained fairly constant at about 1,300 between 1980 and 1997.

Of particular interests for policy makers and social service providers should be the increase in the number of teenage girls involved in delinquency cases. The data indicates that juvenile delinquency caseloads are gender neutral. This is supported by available statistics, which show an increase among female offenders between 1987 and 1996 of 76%, while the increase among males was only 42% (Children's Defense Fund, 2000).

The History of the Juvenile Court System

The juvenile justice system in the United States has a long legacy of focusing on rehabilitation and informality. The creation of a separate juvenile court in 1899 did not change this focus, although it could be argued that it was the beginning of a less formal system for children.

The 1800s provided a glimpse of the social service system in existence today in terms of dealing with delinquent youth. Social organizations, churches, and the social reformers were the key institutions that focused on wayward youth in the era. The role of the government in the oversight of juveniles, at the state or federal level, was minuscule. These organizations and charity groups took the responsibility to establish numerous reform houses, or what were referred to as houses of refuge. These settings were designed to assist young children who found themselves in violation of local laws, by providing them with moral direction and a strong work ethic in hopes of changing their ways. This was also a period when reform schools and foster homes were utilized. The focus of the reform school was on providing a family-like setting with established educational requirements. Similarly, the foster homes were to provide these children with a family like setting, but the key was to place the children in homes away from the city, since the city was viewed as a causal factor in the behavior of the child (Downs and Hess, 2000). As a result of developing these alternative placements for offending youth, adult courts were a viable setting for delinquency hearings because there was little chance of a child receiving an adult sanction.

It is important to note that those who advocated for separate treatment of juveniles did not do so strictly based on their benevolent desires. Although treatment and rehabilitation were believed to be the proper interventions for children with problems, it was also believed these children, most of whom were poor were a threat to the general society. Consequently, the children were subjected to long sentences, intense working hours, and discipline, with the understanding that these children would be cured of their lower class values and develop middle class values and a work ethic (Platt, 1968).

A more systematic approach to delinquency was developed in the late 19th century when the country began to look at more preventive efforts. The YMCA, the YWCA, and other social service organizations began to adopt preventative programming. It was during this period, in 1899, that the Illinois legislature passed the first formal law establishing a juvenile court under its Act to Regulate the Treatment and Control of Dependent, Neglected, and Delinquent Children.

The juvenile court has been defined as "a special court in which children were denied due process and adversarial proceedings in exchange for informal, confidential hearings and dispositions based on what was felt to be in the 'best interest of the child.' It was a court in which distinctions between dependent, neglected, and delinquent children were less important that their common need for state supervision in the manner of a wise and devoted parent" (Schwartz, 1989). Again, this defini-tion points out that the focus was on treatment and rehabilitation, not punishment.

It was not until 1909, during the White House Conference on Youth, that the federal government became officially involved with troubled youth. During this period, courts began to focus on preserving the social order and protecting those with wealth and racial privilege (Krisberg and Austin, 1993). Arguably, things are very similar in today's ap-proach to juvenile justice.

By the early 1950s, every state had adopted a juvenile court and the federal government had instituted legislation to improve conditions for families and children. The most important piece of legislation was the Social Security Act in 1935. It changed the way the nation provided for its most vulnerable and disadvantaged people. The federal government had taken a position on its need to assist citizens and to provide basic needs as well as other supportive services.

The 1960s were a period of radical changes in the politics and life-style of the nation. The civil rights movement dealt with a wide range of individual rights and protections. This included the juvenile justice sys-tem. Between 1960 and 1970, a number of changes occurred in the juve-nile justice system. As the number of youth involved in the juvenile system increased, advocates began to push for more rights. Efforts to decriminalize many of the acts of youth were reassessed. This period brought about a separation of juvenile behaviors into two categories: status offenses and delinquency. The sub category of status offenses re-ferred to behaviors that only a minor could be charged with, i.e., run-away, truant, incorrigible.

There were several key Supreme Court cases that provided expanded rights for juveniles, including: *Kent v. United States*, 1966 (due process in waiver hearings); *In re Gault*, 1967 (notice, counsel, cross examina-tion, and protections against self-incrimination); *In re Winship*, 1970 (standard of proof beyond a reasonable doubt); and *Breed v. Jones*, 1975 (double jeopardy attaches at juvenile adjudication).

During the 1970s the Juvenile Justice and Delinquency Prevention Act of 1974 was passed with two keys goals: deinstitutionalization of status offenses and the separation and removal of juveniles from adult facilities. This act has been amended several times, in 1976, 1977, and 1980 (Drowns and Hess, 2000).

Along with earning more individual protections, the young people involved with the juvenile court also began to see a shift on the treat-ment of youthful offenders. From the late 1970s through the early

1980s, there was a general shift in the attitude toward delinquency and consequently a shift as to the appropriate standard to use—the best interest of the child or the best interest of society. For example, in *Schall v. Martin* (1984), the Supreme Court upheld the right to place juveniles in preventive detention if the youth was perceived as dangerous to themselves or society. This was viewed as a legitimate state interest in protecting society and the juvenile.

Despite the changes in the view of the juvenile justice system and the focus on more punitive treatment, the court remains a less formal and useful option for the less serious offenders.

There are several factors that play into the changes in the juvenile justice system. First, a nation that is fed up with crime and violence and fearful of young people. Second, a political environment that fuels this fear for its own purposes. Finally, the perception of an increase in the number of serious crimes that are being committed in this nation and not just by young people.

Upon review of the history and the changes that have occurred over the past century, two issues come to the forefront: when did the nation stop viewing "delinquent" youth as children, and as alternative approaches are developed to handle juvenile delinquents, how is it determined who and when to use these alternatives?

DOCTRINE OF PARENS PATRIE

The doctrine of Parens Patria refers to the concept that the government will take responsibility for those unable to care for themselves. This doctrine applies to adults as well as children. However, for children, it is the inability or unwillingness of a parent or guardian that will trigger the involvement of the state's role as "parent." This doctrine is pertinent to the discussion because several important questions must be raised concerning the push for punishment versus treatment. What responsibility does the state have in providing for it's troubled youth until the age of majority? Does the state work with them and provide rehabilitative services? Does the state just lock them away?

JUVENILE DELINQUENCY TODAY

The juvenile justice system of today is "not your father's" juvenile justice system. It is much more punitive and focuses less on treatment and rehabilitation. Juveniles under the age of 18 accounted for 26% of the U.S. population and 19% of the total arrests. Much of the attention on young people focuses on the level of violence, including gang and drug related activities (Butts, 1999; Synder and Sickmund, 1999).

Numerous projections forecast that the minority adolescent population will increase significantly by the year 2015. For African Americans, the increase among younger adolescents is expected to increase by about 19%, while for older African American adolescents the increase will be about 21% (Synder and Sickmund, 1999).

The Building Blocks for Youth Initiative confirmed the overrepresentation of African American youth in both the detention population and the population of those transferred from juvenile to adult court. In fact, the report states, "The research demonstrates that minority youth experience a 'cumulative disadvantage' as they move from arrest to referral on charges, to adjudication, and finally to incarceration" (Poe-Yamagata and Jones, 2000).

Disproportionate representation of minorities at every stage of the juvenile justice process is well documented (Synder and Sickmund, 1999). Despite greater awareness and interventions, this situation seems unlikely to be corrected in the near future (Ellis and Sowers, 2000).

As of 1999, minority youth represented 34% of the U. S. population, yet this same group represented 62% of the youth in detention; 67% of the youth committed to public facilities, and 54% of the youth committed to private facilities (Children's Defense Fund, 2000).

The Juvenile Justice and Delinquency Prevention Act of 1974, as originally enacted, included several requirements that primarily addressed custody issues of juveniles. The amendments of 1992 included a section that focused on the overrepresentation and confinement of minority youth, or disproportionate minority confinement. Disproportionate minority confinement (DMC) refers to the point when the proportion of juveniles from minority groups detained or confined in secure detention facilities, secure correctional facilities, jails, and lock ups, exceeds the proportion of such groups as presented in the general population of that state. The DMC mandates that states are to assess reasons for the disproportionate representation of minority youth and to develop strategies to address the causes. However, there is no clear consequence for a failure on the part of the state to comply with the provision aimed at addressing the causes.

TRANSFERS/WAIVERS

The issue of juvenile cases being transferred or waived into adult courts has jolted the juvenile justice system over the past decade. For example, in 1996 there were 47% more delinquency cases waived to criminal court than in 1987. Waivers from juvenile to criminal (adult) court usually include youth charged with serious crimes, as well as those with an extensive juvenile history.

Due to the modifications and changes in many states, the criminal courts now have exclusive or original jurisdiction over juveniles charged with specific crimes. This means that the prosecutor or district attorney can file directly in the criminal court without filing in juvenile court and then seeking a waiver.

The percentage of waivers from juvenile to criminal court has remained relatively constant at about 1.4% since 1985. In 1994, 12,300 juveniles cases were waived by the courts (Downs and Hess, 2000). The numbers are overwhelmingly (95%) males. Although youth under age 15 have seen an increase in the number of waivers from 1987 to 1996, the percentage of those 16 and older has actually fallen from 93% to 88% during this same period (Synder and Sickmund, 1999). It is unclear whether these drops in rates correlate with changes in state laws concerning which courts have original jurisdiction.

The racial disparity in waiver cases is reflective of the general juvenile justice system. The percentage of whites involved in waiver cases decreased during this same period from 57% down to 51%, while the percentage for African Americans increased from 41% to 46%, 44 of whom are African American males (Synder and Sickmund, 1999).

CONCERNS FOR THE AFRICAN AMERICAN COMMUNITY

There are several areas of the juvenile justice system that the African American community must be concerned with: the role that poverty plays into feeding the juvenile justice system; the overrepresentation of Black males; the increase in the number of Black females; and the number of Black victims.

In 1996, African American juveniles represented 30% of all cases in the juvenile justice system, yet only 15% of the general population. Whites were less likely to be detained in secure detention facilities than African American or other minorities, including for drug offenses.

Poverty continues to play a key role in the lives of many urban adolescents. For many children in metropolitan areas, poverty continues to be a major concern. The poverty rate for children under the age of 18 is approximately 20% nationwide. Although children make up only 26% of the population, almost 40% of those in poverty are children under 18.

For the African American community, rates are generally higher. As of 2000, 32% of African American children under the age of 18 were under the poverty level (U.S. Census Bureau, 2000). Although there are no direct correlations between poverty and delinquency, poverty has a number of negative indicators, such as poor health, homelessness, and school failure, which may contribute to anti-social behavior.

As a nation, when discussing the juvenile justice system, there is a tendency to focus on the offenders. Yet, for the African American community, there must also be concern about the victims, since many juveniles become victims of crimes within their schools and neighborhoods. The murder rates for juveniles, which peaked in 1993, in part due to gang warfare nationwide, have declined. However, homicide remains the fourth leading cause of death for children ages 1-4; third for children 5-14; and second for youth 15-24 (Synder and Sickmund, 1999).

IMPLICATIONS

In order to make improvements in the juvenile justice system and to improve relationships with the minority community, several levels of innovative interventions need to be developed.

First, the law enforcement and juvenile justice system must seriously begin to look at the discrepancies that exist in the system and work with the community to develop interactions that are more positive. These institutions must also work with their personnel to address any issues of racial intolerance in order to improve relationships with the minority community. Serious questions need to be addressed concerning the issues of fairness throughout law enforcement and the juvenile justice system.

Second, efforts need to be made to strengthen, not weaken, the Disproportionate Minority Confinement protections of the Juvenile Justice and Delinquency Prevention Act. There have been attempts to weaken current laws, including the Disproportionate Minority Confinement section of the Juvenile Justice and Delinquency Prevention Act, that provide some protection for African American youth. Advocates need to respond to appropriate legislators and community decision-makers about recent reports on juvenile justice and to look closely at a system which overwhelmingly sees minority youth, particularly African American youth, transferred to adult court at astonishingly higher rates than non-minority youth.

Third, involve the Black church, the one institution that has been a consistent strength for the Black community. Recent studies of the impact of religious involvement on adolescents indicate that, for African American youth, religious institutions significantly buffer or interact with the effects of neighborhood disorder on crime, and, in particular, serious crime (Johnson, Jeng et al., 2000). The Black church also assists youth with positive psychosocial development (Markstrom, 1999).

Finally, community based organizations and school systems, working collaboratively, can develop programming directed toward high-risk adolescents. Activities should include academic as well as vocational preparation to help these young people develop the skills necessary to move forward into adulthood. Other interventions could include meaningful and serious programming aimed at early prevention, youth development strategies, the education of police and prosecutors, and most importantly the education of policy makers.

Service providers working with young people, particularly those in prevention programs with high risk or other groups must be aware of the changes in the juvenile/criminal justice system and focus on informing, educating, and advocating to help young people remain outside of the justice system.

Many current interventions with delinquent youth are not developed to specifically meet the needs of African American youth. Instead a one-size fits all intervention is developed, which may or may not be effective for all youth. Race, ethnicity, gender and developmental stage all make important differences in how juveniles view the world and consequently have implications for treatment (Ellis, O'Hara, and Sowers, 1999).

CONCLUSION

Few would disagree with Bilichick (1998) who states that "an effective juvenile justice system must meet three objectives:

1. hold the juvenile offender accountable;
2. enable the juvenile to become a capable, productive, and responsible citizen;
3. ensure safety of the community.

As a nation, we focus on the first and third objectives in Bilichik's statement. It is time to look at how to ensure that objective two can be emphasized. Also missing from these objectives is the right it be fairly treated and accused and not have these critical decision base solely on race and intolerance.

The African American community must challenge its community leaders, politicians, and itself to reassess the direction of the system. Although most would agree that delinquent or criminal behavior must have consequences, it must be done in a fair manner.

TABLE OF CASES

Breed v. Jones, 421 U.S. 519, 5 S. Ct, 1779, 44 L.Ed.2d 346 (1975)

In re Gault, 387 U.S. 1, 87 S. Ct. 1428, 18 L.Ed.2d 527 (1967)

In re Winship, 397 U.S. 358, 90 S. Ct. 1068, 25 L. Ed.2d 368 (1970)

Kent v. United States, 383 U.S. 541, 86 S. Ct. 1045, 16 L. Ed.2d 84 (1966)

Schall v. Martin, 467 U.S. 253, 104 S. Ct. 2403, 81 L. Ed. 2d 207 (1984)

REFERENCES

Bilchik, S. A juvenile justice system for the 21st century. *Crime and Delinquency*, Vol. 44(1), January, 89-101.

Butts, J. (1999). *Youth violence: Perspectives v. reality*. Urban Institute, Presentation to the Board of Trustees.

Children's Defense Fund.(2000). Retrieved March 12, 2001 from the World Wide Web: http://www.childrensdefense.org/ss_violence_jj_quickfacts.htm

Drowns, R. W. and Hess, K. M. (2000). *Juvenile justice*, Belmont, CA: Wadsworth.

Ellis, R. A., O'Hara, M. and Sowers, K.(1999). Treatment profiles of troubled female adolescents: Implications for judicial disposition. *Juvenile and Family Court Journal*, Vol. 50 (3), 25-40.

Ellis, A. and Sowers, K. (2001). *Juvenile justice practice*. Belmont, CA: Wadsworth.

Johnson, B.R., Jeng, S. J., DeLi, S., and Larson, D. (2000). Black youth crises: The church as an agency of local social control, *Journal of Youth and Adolescence*, Vol. 25(4), 479-98.

Juszkiewicz, J. (1999). *Youth crime/adult time: Is justice served*. Washington, D.C.: Building Blocks for Youth.

Krisberg B. and Austin, J. F. (1993). *Reinventing juvenile justice*. Newbury Park, CA: Sage Publications.

Markstrom, C. A. (1999). Religious involvement and adolescent psychological development. *Journal of Adolescence*, 22, 205-225.

Platt, A. (1968). *The child savers: The invention of delinquency*. Chicago, IL: University of Chicago Press.

Poe-Yamagata, E. and Jones, M. A. (2000). *And justice for some: Differential treatment of minority youth in the justice system*. Washington, D.C.: Building Blocks for Youth.

Schwartz, I. M. (1989). *Justice for Juveniles: Re-thinking the best interest of the child.* Lexington, MA: DC & Company.

Synder, H. N. and Sickmund, M. (1999). *Juvenile offenders and victims:1999 national report.* Washington, D.C.: Office of Juvenile Justice and Delinquency Prevention, U.S. Department of Justice.

U.S. Census Bureau. (2000). *Current population survey, Black population in the U.S.: March 2000*, PPL 142.

African American Males at a Crossroad

Stanley F. Battle, MSW, MPH, PhD

SUMMARY. With the recent debates regarding school drop outs, limited parental support, peer pressure, and social isolation, African American males are at a crossroad. For much too long attention has focused on factors that reflect poor self image and a lower sense of control over their destinies. Options are very limited, and it is important to consider the new public policy response to male responsibility utilizing natural support systems. Mentoring is a key variable to establishing greater community responsibility through primary prevention. *[Article copies available for a fee from The Haworth Document Delivery Service: 1-800-HAWORTH. E-mail address: <getinfo@haworthpressinc.com> Website: <http://www.HaworthPress.com> © 2002 by The Haworth Press, Inc. All rights reserved.]*

KEYWORDS. African American males, mentoring, natural support systems

INTRODUCTION

- Almost 90% of persons with AIDS are concentrated in metropolitan areas with populations over 500,000.
- African American men living in Harlem are less likely to reach the age of 65 than men in Bangladesh.
- Fifty-five percent (55%) of all low-income African American, urban children and 16% of all children living in metropolitan areas have lead exposure levels which may result in permanent disability.

Stanley F. Battle is Vice Chancellor of Student and Multicultural Affairs at the University of Wisconsin-Milwaukee.

[Haworth co-indexing entry note]: "African American Males at a Crossroad." Battle, Stanley F. Co-published simultaneously in *Journal of Health & Social Policy (The Haworth Press, Inc.)* Vol. 15, number 2, 2002, pp. 81-91; and: *African-American Adolescents in the Urban Community: Social Services Policy and Practice Interventions* (ed: Judith L. Rozie-Battle) The Haworth Press, Inc., 2002, pp. 81-91. Single or multiple copies of this article are available for a fee from The Haworth Document Delivery Service [1-800-HAWORTH, 9:00 a.m. - 5:00 p.m. (EST). E-mail address: getinfo@haworthpressinc.com].

OVERVIEW

There has probably never been as crucial a time for African American people in the U.S. to begin to define the circumstances, needs, and imperatives of African American family life and the development of African American children as there is now. We are quite aware of the negative perceptions of the African American family. One important aspect of this situation is the occurrence of pregnancy and out-of-wedlock births among African American adolescents, and youth violence. Indeed, the number of single-parent families represents a major concern in the African American community, and unplanned births are at the heart of the issue. Some present conditions that affect the health and well-being of African American families, children, and youth include the steady growth of single-parent households; alarming rates of infant mortality; higher fertility rates, especially among younger adolescents; an increasing percentage of out-of-wedlock births; growing numbers of poor persons and those below the poverty level as defined by the U.S. government; unemployment; and increasingly low levels of family income.

These facts strongly suggest a crisis situation for several reasons. First, effects are multiple and will negatively impact at least two subsequent generations. Second, adequate and effective intervention/prevention techniques have not been utilized to any measurable degree. Descriptive literature and statistical reports have not focused significantly on understanding the interactive, multi-dimensional nature of the situation, especially as it impacts on African American lives. Structural barriers to opportunities, cultural values, and individual coping and adaptive patterns relative to survival and individual development all require academic and community exploration and exposition.

There comes a period in every person's life when the tasks of moving from childhood dependency to adult independence are to be accomplished. Ideally, at this time, a fusion of mental readiness and structural opportunity makes this passage achievable. The continuous and smooth movement of youth from childhood to adulthood, from school to work, from parents' home to one's own home, is essential to the future well-being of both the individual and society. Thus, it is in the interest of society to provide its young people the training (aptitude) and the opportunities (structures) necessary to accomplish these tasks.

Were such conditions optimally available for African American youth, they would be demonstrating a pattern of self-development, at the very least commensurate with that of their White and more likely middle class counterparts. They would be raised in psychologically and economically stable homes, be successful in school, be optimistic about their program and their futures, and successfully transition from school to work. They would, furthermore, as African American youth demonstrate patterns of self-discipline and commitments to self, family and community, reflecting the legacy of struggle for equity and justice of which they are a part. Such does not, however, appear to be the case. Not only do our youth remain "disadvantaged" as compared to other young people, but they are at greater risk than at any other time in recent history. Not only are they being denied structural opportunities, as reflected in the highest high school drop-out and eviction rates, the lowest college attendance, and the well-beyond fifty percent unemployment rates, but African American youth are reflecting alarming attitudinal formations as well.

These youth reflect a lower sense of control over their destinies and an absence of political and collective consciousness, as would unfortunately be expected of children of the post civil rights era. They are subsequently short on mentors and long on rugged individualism. Soaring rates of out-of-wedlock births, "babies having babies" among increasingly younger African American girls with irresponsible and abandoning African American boys, the rising crime and drug abuse rates, and the increasing violence committed by our youth against each other and our elders all speak to a rising despair and declining discipline among our African American youth.

While we recognize the dramatic changes in the American economy and the psychological climate in general that are causal to this shift, we cannot afford to be content with blaming the system and allow an entire generation of our youth to go down the drain. Within this context, an analysis of the state of African-African adolescents and the impact on adolescent African American males follows.

HISTORICAL PORTRAIT
AND THE IMPACT OF SLAVERY

All too often, people ignore Northern slavery and discrimination when revisiting America's past. Although the emancipation war was fought primarily on Southern soil, African Americans around the country suffered the effects of legal and informal racial discrimination. By the seventeenth century, lawmakers had enacted Black codes because "Negroes had become numerous, quarrelsome, and turbulent" (White, 1973). Despite the eventual invalidation of statutory discrimination, African Americans continued to endure the effects of informal socioeconomic oppression as Whites controlled the allocation of resources and opportunities for advancement.

·By 1865, for example, in liberal Hartford, Connecticut, the African American population was estimated at approximately 1,000. Despite their free status (slavery in Connecticut had been phased out decades earlier), African Americans were limited by educational, economic, and political discrimination which was much more covert than that perpetuated against Southern African Americans (Pawlowski, 1973). A 1915 *Hartford Courant* article spoke of Hartford's African American population as a "peaceful and orderly contingent, creating very little trouble in the way of laws . . . generally the people of this race are industrious, happy, and a credit to the city" (Pawlowski, 1973). Such comments revealed the paternalistic attitudes Whites held concerning African Americans and their opinion that African Americans had an accepted place in society.

Two major periods of Northern migration–Pre- and Post-World War I–increased African American populations significantly, as ex-slaves and their descendants fled the South in search of a better living. Despite the presence of various European immigrants in New England, migrant African Americans stood out because of their skin color and slave heritage. As such, any negative activity by African Americans tended to confirm false stereotypes which White residents were all too willing to accept.

As time progressed, major expansion by African Americans throughout the North and to other parts of the city coincided with White flight which was precipitated by the turbulent civil rights era of the 1960s. Thus, many Whites who were opposed to the presence of African Americans in their neighborhoods would often sell their homes to African Americans, as the changing racial composition of various neighborhoods deterred prospective White buyers. Many upwardly-mobile African Americans followed their White counterparts to suburban towns once they achieved a level of economic success. The impact of such flight depleted the resources of the inner city and increased the wealth in surrounding towns. With the migration came a very sober and realistic view of options for African Americans.

CAUSAL FACTORS

Three commonly-cited explanations for African Americans having a greater likelihood to engage in criminal activity are economic deprivation, inadequate socialization, and cultural deviance, all of which are interrelated (Hernstein and Wilson, 1985). African Americans account for a high proportion of the nation's poor. Unemployment is extremely high for men in the 16-30 age group, which also happens to be the same age group responsible for a large share of crime. Although there's no definite cause/effect relationship between economic status and the commission of crime, poor people, many of whom are African American, are more likely to be arrested and incarcerated than nonpoor individuals. Many African Americans, frustrated by actual or perceived lack of opportunities, turn to crime as a means of survival.

Inadequate socialization, a theme popularized by the infamous Moynihan report, proposes that as a result of the legacy of slavery, African American families suffered tremendously and continued to break down, leaving their children ill-equipped to succeed in society. This theme continues to be played out today; however, in its contemporary form, it speaks of declining family values and places blame on individuals rather than on societal conditions which contribute to the continued erosion of the family structure.

The third causal factor, cultural deviance, suggests that African Americans, through the commission of crime and other antisocial acts, are actually resisting against what they perceive as an unjust system. The resulting resentment manifests itself in the expression of violence and deviant behavior. For some, this way of life is learned and becomes entrenched in communities lacking proper resources to combat behavior which is destructive to individuals and the community as a whole.

Such factors fall short of explaining overall tendencies to engage in criminal activity when the range of crimes is expanded to include less visible white-collar crimes. While major white-collar scandals have rocked the nation, White businessmen as a whole have not been characterized as morally debased individuals preying on the weaknesses of others. A convicted White embezzler is likely to be treated less severely by the judicial system than an African American robber who holds up a cab driver for twenty dollars. Although embezzlers steal millions of dollars from investors, their crimes are not perceived to be as serious as those of robbers who threaten physical harm to their victims.

LIFESTYLE DECISIONS: WHAT ARE THE OPTIONS?

When Ronald Reagan declared war on drugs, many were unaware that the casualties of this war would primarily be young, urban African American males. In some states, drug arrests increased by 250% during the 1980s and '90s. For many poor inner-city African American youth, the profits of drug-dealing and the glamorization of the drug culture continue to entice and entrap them in a web of self- and community destruction. While involvement with drugs crosses all racial lines, thousands of urban African Americans continue to be herded into the nation's jails, while others appear to have racial and economic shields which help them to evade capture.

For too many African Americans, especially young males, dealing in drugs offers instant material wealth and improved social standing among peers. Oftentimes, the dealer becomes a role model for others who are impressed by his/her carefree lifestyle, flashy material wealth, and large sums of pocket money. Despite the risks of arrest and violence which accompany involvement in criminal activity, the rewards are too great a lure for those accustomed to doing without. Drug-dealing turns directionless young people into entrepreneurs. For many, it's a lifestyle from which they can't return, as the financial rewards become addictive and irreplaceable.

Some family members and friends of drug dealers quietly condone the dealer's activities despite their own noninvolvement. Often the young African American drug dealer becomes a major economic contributor to the family's resources. The following statement by "Joe" (not his real name), a 17-year-old African American male who sells drugs, illustrates this point: "My family (mother and siblings) knows how I make money but they don't sweat me too much because I look out for them. It's something I gotta do 'cause there ain't no jobs out there." For some families, the drug-dealing son replaces the father who, if present, would be expected to be the major economic provider in the family.

The addict is like the prostitute for the pimp, as he or she sacrifices his or her body for the dealer's gain. Often referred to as "pagers" because of their frequent contacts via beeper with the dealer, the addict will go to any extreme to support his or her habit. Loyal customers and expansion of clientele are the main goals of the dealer. Good will is extremely important, for having a reputation of treating customers right by providing them with a worthy product will ensure their return and attract new business.

The most popular drugs on the streets from the dealers' perspectives are cocaine and heroin, as they offer the greatest profits in the shortest amount of time. This is due largely to the effects of both drugs, which provide the user with intense highs and subsequent crashes. In order to avoid the trauma associated with crashing, the craving addict or "fiend" is only concerned with getting more drugs to maintain a high and a sense of euphoria. Marijuana use is also very popular and is viewed by some as a safe alternative to hardcore drugs.

Children of drug-dependent persons are often neglected to the point where they end up being cared for by relatives, friends, or being placed in foster care or other state institutions. Many of these same children will themselves be vulnerable to the lure of drug use and/or dealing. Babies born to addicted women often suffer major physical problems. Other effects of drugs on the community include an increase in the spread of the AIDS virus as a result of adults sharing dirty needles and having multiple sexual partners. While condom distribution and dispensing of clean needles has occurred in several cities, it is unlikely craving addicts are able to fully appreciate risks during a drug-induced state.

In his book, *When Work Disappears: The World of the New Urban Poor*, William Julius Wilson talks about a time during segregation when there were jobs in the community. Now in the 1990s in African American communities, there are few jobs. We are not part of the information superhighway because we lack hard skills.

YOUTH VIOLENCE

Most people are aware of the fact that homicide is the leading natural cause of death for African American males aged 15-24 years. Nationally, juvenile arrest rates increased 89% between 1980 and 1990. These statistics cry out for remediation as many residents, especially youth, live under conditions which greatly enhance their chance of being victims of violent crime.

Reasons offered for the explosion in youth violence include the continued breakdown of the American family, easy availability of guns, the eroding quality of public schools, and the glorification of violence in the media (Butterfield, 1992). According to a study by the National Crime Analysis Project at Northeastern University (the results of which appeared in a 1992 *New York Times* article), there has been a 24% increase in homicides nationwide, and a 36% increase in overall violent crime, due largely to an unexpected surge of violence among young boys.

A local violence prevention program strongly recommends that youth violence–primarily viewed as a criminal problem–should be understood as a public health problem which can be prevented by teaching adolescents how to identify factors leading to violence, as well as positive nonviolent conflict resolution strategies (Lang, 1992). For children, such efforts are greatly needed as children are twice as likely to be murdered today as those from their parents' generation.

All too often, youth violence is blamed solely on the drug epidemic and gang activity; such short-sighted approaches ignore the issue of adult responsibility.

NEW PUBLIC POLICY RESPONSE: MALE RESPONSIBILITY THROUGH NATURAL SUPPORT SYSTEMS

For several decades, the United States has led all developed Western countries in rates of teenage pregnancy and childbearing. While the extent of teenage parenthood in this country remains significant, the rate of births to teens has been declining since the 1970s for the most part because of the increased availability of contraceptives and abortion. In spite of this decline, adolescent childbearing has become one of the most pressing issues facing our society because births to teens are increasingly births to unmarried teens.

CASE EXAMPLE: NEW APPPROACH IN MILWAUKEE: MENTORING BOYS TO MEN

Many approaches have been tried, but this one requires personal sacrifice and a commitment of the most valuable commodity we have–time. Men from four major ethnic groups will be recruited to work together and mentor boys.

There has probably never been as crucial a time for African Americans, Latino, Caribbean, and Native American people in the United States to begin to define the circumstances, needs, and imperatives of family life in our communities. The effort to mentor boys in Milwaukee, Wisconsin has a goal of reaching 1,000 boys and mentors on a one-to-one level.

In Milwaukee, as in many other urban cities across the country, one will quickly notice that in too many instances, the adult male is missing. The minority male has too often fallen victim to discrimination and economic castration.

In short, we are fighting to overcome what Ralph Ellison writes about in *The Invisible Man*–the man with limited access and the man who is not understood.

Mission

The mission of this initiative is threefold:

1. to secure an appropriate match for boys who are African American, Hispanic, and Native American–ages 5-9, 10-13, and 14-18;
2. to create an environment where African American, Hispanic, and Native American men can work together on saving minority boys,
3. to provide support for single parents who are frequently women. In addition, professional support will be available to mentors and parents by tracking the matches. Mentors will participate in extensive training.

Special Features of the Program

The first priority is to match our mentors and mentees. This relationship will grow out of role modeling, respect, honesty, and cultural diversity. Second, a strong working relationships between men who are African American, Hispanic, and Native American will be built. Young minority boys statistically lead in all of the major categories for poor outcomes in health and the percentage of males who are incarcerated. Men of color must support their youth and each other. Third, and the most important, there will be support single parents, with a special focus on the mother. The single parent of the mentee will work closely with the staff and mentor to help address problems in their life. The mentor/mentee's relationship is only one part of the equation. The mentor/mentee relationship cannot solve all the problems in the family, but it can help. In addition, with assistance from staff and the mentors, positive relief will be provided in the lives of many young men.

Basics for Success

Mentor Recruitment

Unlike many methods of finding people to fill positions, the initiative will take a very unusual approach to finding the special person needed as a mentor. Because of the uniqueness of the program and the special needs of our population, the mentors must be special individuals.

The main resource will be support staff and community contacts, which include churches, schools, one-on-one meetings with people who are personally known in the community, and support from local community-based agencies. Each person referred to the program must be recommended by a responsible member of the community before they will be considered as a potential member. There is a good chance that a large number of potential members may be missed, but the process feels more comfortable because it is homegrown, yet still has all the necessary ingredients required to be very professional. Each mentor will be interviewed by the support staff and police checks will be done. Mentors and mentees from similar racial backgrounds will be matched.

The media outlets to be utilized include the following:

- broadcast radio and television;
- public service announcements that identify the program, its benefits to participants, and a contact person (address and phone number) from whom additional information can be obtained;
- disseminate program information through churches and other community-based organizations within each of the target schools and communities;
- advertise the program in community newspapers; and
- face-to-face contact will be made by support staff with mentees and parents to explain the program benefits and responsibilities, and address any concerns they may have.

Selection of Mentees

Mentees will be selected from the Metropolitan Milwaukee area. In addition, visits will be made to the elementary, middle, and high schools to insure that students are familiar with the program. Natural support systems will be utilized, including churches, barber shops, and community agencies. The goal is to do nation building for the mentors and the boys. At this point, there really is no need to expect someone else to do it.

This is a joint partnership with Opportunities for Industrialization Center of Greater Milwaukee and the Sullivan-Spaights Professor at the University of Wisconsin-Milwaukee.

CONCLUSION

There are no quick fixes and we cannot afford to moralize young males. A concerted effort is required to address the needs of parenting males, especially concerning the problems of unemployment and education. However, attention must be paid to the total population of males at risk. Solutions must be realistic and focus on how society should address the needs of adolescents and children. Senator Daniel Patrick Moynihan proposed that a national policy be developed that would treat families with children (including males) the way we treat the elderly, that is, with provisions for income indexing and tax breaks. But the track record with the elderly has been poor, and young people do not have a strong political base, to ensure they would fare any better.

Education, prevention, and community responsibility are the key ingredients to dealing with the needs of African American males. Such education must include parents, teachers, community members, and teenagers. Prevention goes hand in hand with exposure to appropriate information that includes sex education, accessibility to contraceptives, educational and career options, and access to appropriate role models. Adult males who work 40-60 hours per week and provide for their families are excellent role models. One does not have to be a film star or professional athlete to be a role model. The many strengths that already exist in the African American community must be utilized.

Community health care clinics can play an important role in providing education and counseling in sexuality, family planning, health/nutrition, and life options. Further, community groups can assist with career counseling, employment training, and job placement. Success is measured in terms of education and a job. Thus, with appropriate exposure, young males will be able to make appropriate decisions and become self-sufficient.

I am an invisible man. . . . I am a man of substance, of flesh and bone, fiber and liquids–and I might even be said to possess a mind. I am invisible, understand, simply because people refuse to see me. . . . When they approach me, they see only my surroundings, themselves, or figments of their imagination–indeed, everything and anything except me.

–Ralph Ellison (1972), *Invisible Man*

REFERENCES

Butterfield, F. (1992). Seeds of murder epidemic: Teenage boys with guns. *New York Times*, October 19, A8.

Ellison, R.(1995). *The invisible man*. 2nd edition. New York, NY: Vintage Books/Random House.

Hernstein, R. and Wilson, J.(1985). *Crime and nature*. New York: Simon and Shuster.

Lang, J. (1992). Viewing youth violence as a health problem. *The Hartford Courant*, September 20, 8.

Pawlowski, R. (1973). *How the other half lived: An ethnic history of the old east side south end of Hartford, Connecticut*.

White, P. (1973). *Connecticut's black soldier*, Chester, CT: Pequot Press.

Wilson, J. W. (1997). *When work disappears: The world of the new urban poor*. New York, NY: Vintage Books/Random House.

Index

Academy for Education
    Development, 20
Act to Regulate the Treatment and
    control of Dependent,
    Neglected, and Delinquent
    Children, 71
Adoption and Safe Families Act
    (ASFA), 7
African American adolescents. *See*
    Changing school
    environment; Health
    concerns for youth; Males at
    a crossroad; Neo-juvenile
    justice system; Teen fathers,
    child support issues and;
    Teenage girls, challenges
    faced by; Youth development
    strategy; Youth in the new
    millennium
After-School Initiative (ASI), 18
AIDS. *See* HIV/AIDS
Alcohol abuse, 40-41
America's Promise, 21
Annie E. Casey Foundation, 36,37
ASFA (Adoption and Safe Families
    Act, 7
ASI (After-School Initiative), 18

Battle, Stanley, 35,81
Big Brothers/Big Sisters, 21
Breed v. *Jones,* 72,78
Building Blocks for Youth Initiative, 74

Carnegie Council on Adolescent
    Development, 14

Center for Early Adolescence, 14
Center for Youth Development, 14
Changing school environment, 26-27
    African American student struggle
        academic success
            misconceptions, 29
        "cool" personality
            characteristics, 29-30
        culturally relevant teaching,
            30-31
        not "acting White" concept, 30
        student empowerment, 30,32
    Fourth Grade Failure Syndrome,
        26,31
    implications and recommendations
        regarding, 31-32
    summary regarding, 25
    teacher centered classrooms, 26-27
    teacher expectations, 31
    traditional school system
        analytical *vs.* relational learning
            styles, 28,31
        curriculum, 27-28
        dominant culture values, 27-28
        school culture, 28-29
        teacher, student statistics, 27
        verbal-linguistic teaching methods,
            26,27,28-29
    winning identity formula concept,
        26,32
Child support. *See* Teen fathers, child
        support issues and
Child Support Distribution Act, 51
Child welfare, 10
    foster care, 7
    kinship care, 7
    legislation regarding, 7
    statistics regarding, 6,7

See also Teen fathers, child support issues and
Cocaine abuse, 40
Comer, James, 15,22
Communities
  changes in, 15
  positive youth development strategies, 17-19,21
  violence in, 6
Crack cocaine abuse, 40

DeWitt Wallace Reader's Digest Fund, 14,20
Disproportionate minority confinement (DMC), 74,76
DMC. *See* Disproportionate minority confinement
Drug abuse, increase in, 14

Education
  entrance exam scores and, 9
  oppositional attitudes towards, 8
  statistics regarding, 8
  See also Changing school environment
Education and Youth Development Policy, Research and Advocacy program (National Urban League), 20
Ellison, Ralph, 88,91

Failure, effects of, 3
Family structure
  extended family networks and, 5
  peer groups, youth gangs, 5
  religious affiliation, 5
  statistics regarding, 5
Family Support Act of 1988, 50
Foster care
  kinship care, 7
  statistics regarding, 7
Fourth Grade Failure Syndrome, 26

Gangs, 14
  See also Violence
Genetic inferiority theory of youth violence, 3

Head Start, 19
  Health concerns for youth
  health care gaps, 36
  health institutions, relationships with, 43
  health insurance, 41-42, 43*table*
  high risk behavior, 35
  sexually transmitted diseases (STDs), 38-40
  substance abuse, 40-41
    alcohol and drug relationship, 40-41
    crack cocaine epidemic, 40
    Monitoring the Future (MTF) Study, 41
    trend changes, 40
  summary regarding, 35,43-44
  teen pregnancies, 17
    birth control methods, 37
    HIV/AIDS issues, 37-38
    short term interventions, 38
    statistics regarding, 36,37
    teen attitudes, 37
Health insurance
  managed care organizations, impact of, 42
  statistics regarding, 41-42,43*table*
HIV/AIDS
  sexually transmitted diseases and, 39
  statistics regarding, 81
  teen pregnancies, 37-38

In re Gault, 72,78
In re Winship, 72,78
Incentives to Excel and Succeed (National Urban League), 18

Institutional racism, 4
Invisible Man (Ellison), 88,91

Justice system. *See* Neo-juvenile
    justice system
Juvenile Justice and Delinquency
    Prevention Act, 72,74,76
Juvenile justice system, 10 *See also*
    Neo-juvenile justice system

Kent v. *United States,* 72,78
Kinship care, 7

Males at a crossroad
    African American family trends, 82
    causal factors, 84-85
    cultural deviance, 84,85
    drug dealing, 85-87
    male responsibility, 81,88
    mentoring boys to men, 88,89-90
        mentee selection, 90
        mentor recruitment, 89-90
        mission, 89
        program features, 89
    natural support systems, 81,88,90
    poverty factors, 83,84,85
    slavery, impact of, 83-84
    socialization inadequacies, 84,85
    summary regarding, 81,91-92
    youth to adult transitions, 82-83
    youth violence, 87-88
A Matter of Time (Comer), 15
Medical Expenditure Panel Survey
    (MEPS), 42
Mentoring, 21-22,88
    mentee selection, 90
    mentor recruitment, 89-90
    mission, 89
    program features, 89
MEPS. *See* Medical Expenditure Panel
    Survey

Milwaukee, Wisconsin. *See* Mentoring
Monitoring the Future (MTF) Study,
    41
Mott Foundation, 14

National Conference of
    Commissioners on Uniform
    State Laws (NCCUSL),
    49,51
National Urban League, Education and
    Youth Development Policy,
    Research and Advocacy
    program, 20
National Urban League's Incentives to
    Excel and Succeed
    (NULITES), 18
NCCUSL (National Conference of
    Commissioners on Uniform
    State Laws), 49,51
Neo-juvenile justice system
    Black church community, 77
    confidentiality of court records, 70
    court cases regarding, 78
    crime rate trends, 69-70,74
    disproportionate minority
        confinement (DMC),
        74,75,76
    gender factors, 70,75
    history of, 70-73
        civil rights movement, 72
        1800s, 71
        federal government role, 72
        juvenile court, defined, 71-72
        social service organizations, 71
        Supreme Court cases, 72
        youthful offender treatment,
        72-73
    implications regarding, 76-77
    juvenile victims, 76
    juvenile *vs.* adult status, 70,74-75
    Parens Patrie doctrine, 73
    policing policies, 69
    poverty issues, 75-76
    punishment policies, 69,73-74

rehabilitation trends, 69
summary regarding, 69,77-78
transfers, waivers, 74-75
NULITES (National Urban League's
    Incentives to Excel and
    Succeed), 18

Parens Patria doctrine, 73
Personal Responsibility and Work
    Opportunity Reconciliation
    Act (PRWORA), 7,50-51
Positive youth development (PYD)
    concept
    non-events focus of, 16
    positive assets of youth, 16
Post Traumatic Stress Disorder (PTSD),
    domestic violence and, 6
Poverty
    culture of poverty theory, youth
        violence and, 3,10
    juvenile justice system, 75-76
    male decision making, 83,84,85
    statistics regarding, 4-5
    teenage girls, 64
PRWORA (Personal Responsibility
    and Work Opportunity
    Reconciliation Act), 7,50-51
PTSD (Post Traumatic Stress
    Disorder), 6
PYD (positive youth development)
    concept, 16-17

Racial discrimination
    institutional racism, 4
    youth violence theory of, 3
Revised Uniform Reciprocal
    Enforcement of Support Act
    (RURESA), 50
Rozie-Battle, Judith, 1,13,45,69
RURESA (Revised Uniform
    Reciprocal Enforcement of
    Support Act), 50

Schall v. *Martin,* 73,78
Schools. *See* Changing school
    environment
Search Institute, 14
Sexually transmitted diseases (STDs)
    description of, 37-38
    statistics regarding, 39-40
Smith, Sabra R., 25
Social Security Act, 1935, 72
Social services. *See* Child welfare
STDs. *See* Sexually transmitted
    diseases
Stoneman, Dorothy, 38
Strive Media Institute (Strive), 18-19
Students. *See* Changing school
    environment
Substance abuse
    alcohol and drug relationship, 40-41
    crack cocaine epidemic, 40
    Monitoring the Future (MTF)
        Study, 41
    trend changes, 40
Sullivan-Spaights Boys to Men
    Mentoring Institute, 21

TANF (Temporary Assistance to
    Needy Families), 46
Technology advancements, urban
    youth and, 1-2
Teen fathers, child support issues and
    community education programs, 55
    developmental status of father, 51-52
    drop-out rates, 45
    father's rights, 46
    financial focus, 47-48
    "grandparent liability," 52
    job training programs, 55
    legislation to enforce, 49-51,52
    paternity, 46-47
        defined, 46
    paternity adjudication, 46
    policy implications of
        in-kind contributions, 54
        prevention programs, 54

prejudicial social factors, 52
prevention programs, 54-56
role of fathers, 47-49
safety issues, 48
summary regarding, 45-46,56
"tender years doctrine," 47
unemployment rates, 45,53,54
Teen pregnancies, 17
birth control methods, 37
HIV/AIDS issues, 37-38
short term interventions, 38
statistics regarding, 14,36,37
teen attitudes, 37
Teenage girls, challenges faced by, 60
crime and gangs, 64
family demographics, 64-65
family functioning, impact of, 61-62
implications regarding, 64-66
peer pressure, 60,64
poverty rates, 64
resiliency, 62-63
role of the church, 60,63-64,65
self-esteem, 61-62,65
STDs, 60
substance abuse, 60
summary regarding, 59,66
unemployment rates, 65
violence against, 60
White beauty images, 62
See also Teen pregnancies
Temporary Assistance to Needy
Families (TANF), 46

UIFSA (Uniform Interstate Family
Support Act), 50
Uniform Interstate Family Support Act
(UIFSA), 50
Uniform Parentage Act (UPA), 51
Uniform Reciprocal Enforcement of
Support Act (URESA), 49-50
UPA (Uniform Parentage Act), 51
URESA (Uniform Reciprocal
Enforcement of Support Act),
49-50

Violence
domestic violence, 6
effects of, 3
increase in, 14
male decision-making and, 87-88
peak hours of, 20
in schools, community, 6
See also Gangs

Washington, Booker T., 32
*When Teens Have Sex: Issues and
Trends* (Annie E. Casey
Foundation), 37

Youth Development Community
Block Grant Bill (HR 2807),
20
Youth development strategy, 17-18
adolescent cohort, needs of, 15
church programs, 21
community strategies, 13,17-19,21
community support, decrease in, 15
early childhood interventions,
14-15
extended family support, 15-16
importance of, 13-16,17-19
long term programming and
services, 19-20
media participation, 21-22
mentoring programs, 21-22
middle through high school years,
19-20
national youth organizations, 14,
18-19
non-events focus of, 16
participation of youth in, 17
policy recommendations,
implications, 19-22
school and community programs,
14
social competence facilitation,
17-18

summary regarding, 13,22
violence, increase in, 14
youth work and workers, 20-21
Youth in the new millenium
    alienation of, 2
    antisocial behavior and, 2-3
    child welfare, 6-7,10
    church support, 5
    community violence, 6
    culture of poverty theory and, 3
    education, 7-9
    extended family support, 5-6
    failure and, effects of, 3
    family structure and supports, 5-6,9
    genetic inferiority theory and, 3
    "hip-hop" generation, 2-4

implications regarding, 9-10
institutional racism and, effects of,
    4
juvenile justice system, 10
oppositional culture concept and,
    4,9
peer groups, youth gangs, 5
poverty statistics, 4-5
racial discrimination theory and, 3
summary regarding, 1,10
technology advancements, 1-2
violence exposure, effects of, 3
Youth Risk Behavior Surveillance
    Study, 41
YouthBuild U.S.A., 38